T0073924

Madness in the Family

STUDIES OF THE WEATHERHEAD EAST ASIAN INSTITUTE, COLUMBIA UNIVERSITY

The Studies of the Weatherhead East Asian Institute of Columbia University were inaugurated in 1962 to bring to a wider public the results of significant new research on modern and contemporary East Asia.

Selected Titles

(Complete list at: https://weai.columbia.edu/studies-weatherhead-east-asian-institute/)

The Sound of Salvation: Voice, Gender, and the Sufi Mediascape in China, by Guangtian Ha. Columbia University Press, 2022.

Carbon Technocracy: Energy Regimes in Modern East Asia, by Victor Seow. University of Chicago Press, 2022.

Disunion: Anticommunist Nationalism and the Making of the Republic of Vietnam, by Nu-Anh Tran. University of Hawai'i Press, 2022.

Learning to Rule: Court Education and the Remaking of the Qing State, 1861–1912, by Daniel Barish. Columbia University Press, 2022.

Policing China: Street-Level Cops in the Shadow of Protest, by Suzanne Scoggins. Cornell University Press, 2021.

Mobilizing Japanese Youth: The Cold War and the Making of the Sixties Generation, by Christopher Gerteis. Cornell University Press, 2021.

Middlemen of Modernity: Local Elites and Agricultural Development in Modern Japan, by Christopher Craig. University of Hawai'i Press, 2021.

Isolating the Enemy: Diplomatic Strategy in China and the United States, 1953–1956, by Tao Wang. Columbia University Press, 2021.

A Medicated Empire: The Pharmaceutical Industry and Modern Japan, by Timothy M. Yang. Cornell University Press, 2021.

Dwelling in the World: Family, House, and Home in Tianjin, China, 1860–1960, by Elizabeth LaCouture. Columbia University Press, 2021.

Made in Hong Kong: Transpacific Networks and a New History of Globalization, by Peter Hamilton. Columbia University Press, 2021.

China's Influence and the Center–Periphery Tug of War in Hong Kong, Taiwan and Indo-Pacific, by Brian C. H. Fong, Wu Jieh-min, and Andrew J. Nathan. Routledge, 2020.

The Power of the Brush: Epistolary Practices in Chosŏn Korea, by Hwisang Cho. University of Washington Press, 2020.

On Our Own Strength: The Self-Reliant Literary Group and Cosmopolitan Nationalism in Late Colonial Vietnam, by Martina Thucnhi Nguyen. University of Hawaiʻi Press, 2020.

A Third Way: The Origins of China's Current Economic Development Strategy, by Lawrence Chris Reardon. Harvard University Asia Center, 2020.

Disruptions of Daily Life: Japanese Literary Modernism in the World, by Arthur M. Mitchell. Cornell University Press, 2020.

Recovering Histories: Life and Labor after Heroin in Reform-Era China, by Nicholas Bartlett. University of California Press, 2020.

Figures of the World: The Naturalist Novel and Transnational Form, by Christopher Laing Hill. Northwestern University Press, 2020.

Arbiters of Patriotism: Right Wing Scholars in Imperial Japan, by John Person. University of Hawaiʻi Press, 2020.

Making It Count: Statistics and Statecraft in the Early People's Republic of China, by Arunabh Ghosh. Princeton University Press, 2020.

Tea War: A History of Capitalism in China and India, by Andrew B. Liu. Yale University Press, 2020.

MADNESS
IN THE FAMILY

Women, Care, and Illness in Japan

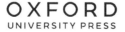

H. YUMI KIM

OXFORD

UNIVERSITY PRESS

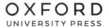

Oxford University Press is a department of the University of Oxford. It furthers
the University's objective of excellence in research, scholarship, and education
by publishing worldwide. Oxford is a registered trade mark of Oxford University
Press in the UK and certain other countries.

Published in the United States of America by Oxford University Press
198 Madison Avenue, New York, NY 10016, United States of America.

CIP data is on file at the Library of Congress
ISBN 978–0–19–750735–3

DOI: 10.1093/oso/9780197507353.001.0001

This book was published with the assistance of the Association for
Asian Studies (AAS) First Book Subvention Program.

For my parents, Jongchun and Stella Kim

Contents

Acknowledgments

COMPLETING A BOOK about women and their caregiving labor during the ongoing COVID-19 pandemic has been both unsettling and illuminating. This labor is often taken for granted, its effects on the mental health of women and their families rendered invisible to the public eye. In such a moment, it feels especially necessary and urgent to acknowledge the intellectual, mental, and emotional labors of the various people who have helped shape this book.

The seeds of this project were sown at Columbia University, where Carol Gluck and Kim Brandt served as model historians and mentors. They gave me free range to explore and grow on my own terms, stepping in with incisive feedback at crucial moments. Matthew Jones, Betsy Blackmar, Gregory Pflugfelder, and David Lurie shared invaluable insights. Elsewhere, Andreas Killen (CUNY) guided me through comparative studies of mental illness, and Alan Tansman (UC Berkeley) always asked the obvious questions that had no obvious answers. Support from the Weatherhead East Asian Institute, the Jerrold Seigel Fellowship in Cultural and Intellectual History, and the Mellon Graduate Fellowship at the Interdisciplinary Center for Innovative Theory and Empirics, with Bill McAllister at the helm, provided financial and moral support, as well as an office I could call my own.

In Japan, a dynamic community of scholars welcomed me with generosity and kindness. Suzuki Akihito, then at Keio University and now at the University of Tokyo, graciously offered much of his time and support during my first extended stay in Tokyo. He continues to help with matters both big and small, for which I am ever grateful. Hashimoto Akira at Aichi Prefectural University guided me toward important sources and kindly invited me to present at workshops on the history of psychiatry. Itahara Kazuko of Osaka University of Health and Sport Sciences organized my visit to Eitokuji in Osaka, which shaped the first chapter of this book and my broader interests in cultures of health and healing. Hyōdō Akiko, whose scholarship has long inspired my own, was generous with her time and energy. Okamoto Kōichi at

Waseda University kindly sponsored me as an exchange researcher. Support from a Fulbright IIE Fellowship defrayed the costs of research and living in Japan.

At Johns Hopkins University, my colleagues in the Department of History have offered unparalleled support and inspiration. Special thanks to Tobie Meyer-Fong, who has provided sustenance in many forms from the moment I stepped on campus. François Furstenberg has been unstintingly helpful and generous. Bill Rowe, Michael Kwass, Nathan Connolly, Erin Rowe, Todd Shepard, Ken Moss, Angus Burgin, and John Marshall have been extraordinarily supportive, as have Casey Lurtz, Jessica Marie Johnson, Liz Thornberry, Katie Hindmarch-Watson, and Tamer el-Leithy. I thank all my departmental colleagues for setting the bar so wonderfully high. In the Program in East Asian Studies, as well as the Department of the History of Medicine, I have found community and camaraderie. I especially thank Clara Han and Erin Chung for their help in putting out some fires, while stoking others, when necessary. Their brilliance and savvy continue to guide me, both professionally and personally. My writing partner extraordinaire Mary Fissell read countless versions of this book, never failing to say exactly what I needed to hear. Marta Hanson, Rebecca Brown, Yulia Frumer, Elizabeth O'Brien, and Jeremy Greene have helped me in the final stages of writing. The Japan Foundation sponsored a book conference, where a group of Hopkins colleagues and two external readers guided the manuscript toward completion. I am deeply grateful for Sabine Frühstück's perceptive comments, as well as Jordan Sand's discerning readings. Both helped me better understand what I wanted to say in the book. Support from the David B. Larson Fellowship at the John W. Kluge Center in the Library of Congress enabled me to finish the research for this book, while also laying the groundwork for future work.

Friends and colleagues who have crisscrossed Tokyo, New York City, Berkeley, and Baltimore with me have provided generative and nourishing conversations throughout the years. Alyssa Park and Jenny Wang Medina—my gratitude for their humor, brilliance, and humility is endless. A group of fellow mom-scholars have buoyed me throughout many years: Sayaka Chatani, Gal Gvili, Chelsea Szendi Schieder, Liza Lawrence, Mi-Ryong Shim, Stacey Van Fleet, and Yurou Zhong. Many years ago, a fortuitous encounter in Tokyo enabled me to meet Maiko Morimoto, who helped so much in the earliest stages of this project that I could write a separate acknowledgment just for her. Gabe Paquette and Johanna Richlin helped make Baltimore a warm and welcoming place for our family. For their intellectual and moral support, I also thank David Atherton, Kyoungjin Bae, Joshua Batts, Emily

Baum, Claudia Cameron, Caleb Carter, Anna Clark, BuYun Chen, Divya Cherian, Andre Deckrow, Chad Diehl, Arunabh Ghosh, Shinhee Han, Lisa Hofmann-Kuroda, Michelle Hwang, Colin Jones, Jon Kief, Minjae Kim, George Lazopoulos, Rev. Seunghyun Lee, Sungyun Lim, Tatiana Linkhoeva, Andy Liu, Andrew Leong, Patrick Luhan, Daryl Maude, Jennie Miller, Ti Ngo, Patrick Noonan, Paul Roquet, Luke Thompson, Jim Wilkinson, Tim Yang, and Christina Yi.

Librarians, archivists, and staff across several institutions provided invaluable assistance, including Shimizu Fusako at the Komine Institute in Tokyo; Toshie Marra at the C. V. Starr East Asian Library at the University of California, Berkeley; Eiichi Ito in the Asian Division at the Library of Congress; and the staff of the National Diet Library in Japan. At Johns Hopkins, librarian Yunshan Ye and curator Lael Ensor-Bennett at the Visual Resources Collection provided invaluable (and prompt!) assistance. My research assistants Yuri Amano, Hannah Lee Scherr, and Nandini Dey stepped in at the eleventh hour to ensure that the final details were in order.

I am grateful to have met Susan Ferber at Oxford University Press, who skillfully guided this project through its various stages. Two readers for the Press offered valuable suggestions, which I hope I have successfully incorporated into the final product.

My family has sustained me with tremendous love and support through this long process. My parents, Jongchun and Stella Kim, and their lifelong commitment to the public good inspired me to write about how people care for one another in difficult times. My sister, Bouree Kim, who has dedicated her professional life to supporting survivors of trauma and loss, has shown unconditional support. Her advice to write the book that I did not think I could write proved invaluable. My husband, Alex Kwon, has been my anchor in what were often rough seas. I thank him for always reminding me of what matters most. Joongbin and Ahmi, both of whom entered the world as I wrote and re-wrote the book, are my everlasting sources of brightness. They are also my greatest teachers. Without them, I would not know the profound and layered realities of what it means to care.

Madness in the Family

Introduction

IN A VILLAGE tucked away in the remote mountains of southwestern Japan, a young woman begins to babble about fried tofu and red beans, widely known as the favored foods of foxes. She rubs her nose and paces back and forth. Distressed by their daughter's unusual behavior, her mother and father summon a local religious healer to exorcise what they surmise is the spirit of a fox that clings to her body—but to no avail. The year is 1891, and one of the nation's first European-trained psychiatrists is beginning to travel from Tokyo to this rural village and others in the region, famous for their cases of "fox attachment" (*kitsune tsuki*), or the overtaking of human minds and bodies by fox spirits. Although the psychiatrist and local officials try to convince the family that their daughter suffers not from the workings of a fox spirit but from "mental illness" (*seishinbyō*, literally "sickness of spirit"), the new diagnosis proves unhelpful. Not only is the term strange and unfamiliar, but there are no nearby doctors or facilities to treat such illnesses. When the daughter begins to wander into the backwoods, the family fears she may inflict harm upon herself and their neighbors and decides that they have no choice but to confine her in a makeshift cage built inside their house. Such a solution was a long-standing custom across the country for the safeguarding of the mentally disturbed and those around them.

After a few weeks of confinement, the daughter's condition improves enough that the family dismantles the cage and the household returns to its usual rhythms. By 1910 she has married and moved to Osaka, a sprawling city with over 1 million residents. She and her family have most likely kept the fox-spirit attachment and caging a secret, since her in-laws would not have approved the marriage had they known. Still, her new family, especially her mother-in-law, readily finds reasons for reproach. The young woman has not given birth to any children, tires easily, and sulks over minor mishaps. Feeling

Madness in the Family. H. Yumi Kim, Oxford University Press. © Oxford University Press 2022.
DOI: 10.1093/oso/9780197507353.003.0001

despondent, she might glance at newspaper and magazine advertisements for patent medicines to treat what experts call "women's diseases," typically conditions that affected fertility. When she begins experiencing convulsions, her husband and mother-in-law decide that an expert opinion is necessary. Taking advantage of a city with a booming marketplace of mental and spiritual healing, they first take her to a gynecologist and then a psychiatric rest home, where she stays for a week. But the convulsions persist. Neither the treatment of a famed religious healer nor bed rest helps. Finally, her mother-in-law and husband send her back to her parents' home in the countryside, returning her to the setting in which the first signs of her affliction appeared. The babbling begins anew, except this time she mumbles not about fried tofu and red beans, but about unborn babies and suspicious neighbors.

The story of this unnamed young woman is a composite of several accounts of actual Japanese women who suffered from various forms of mental and spiritual affliction from the 1880s to 1930s.[1] Her narrative conveys what the historical archive has tended to obscure: the ongoing centrality of family in the care of those considered mad and in the creation of gendered understandings of madness. Journals, newspapers, books, advertisements, and other print media from the turn of the twentieth century would suggest that the management of the so-called mad or mentally ill had shifted from family members to the European-trained Japanese psychiatrists. Trained abroad in Germany and in new state-sponsored and private medical schools in Japan, the first Japanese psychiatrists began conducting original research, publishing journals, and building asylums in the 1880s. By the 1900s, at least one public asylum, along with many private mental hospitals, dotted the therapeutic landscape of major cities across the country. Outside asylum walls, psychiatrists promoted hospital-based care in discussions about crime, pathology, sexuality, and mental hygiene in national newspapers and magazines, finding platforms for their ideas in popular culture and securing a place in the criminal justice system. Psychiatry became known as the site of some of the most cutting-edge developments in the treatment of madness.

But while psychiatric institutions and doctors occupied the public spotlight, the majority of afflicted individuals remained in the care and custody of their families. Family members were the first to observe and diagnose the behavior of one of their own as strange or otherwise inexplicable. Even for families who could afford to send their relative to one of the new psychiatric hospitals, they would have already identified the causes of her suffering, drawing on vocabularies of madness specific to time and place, as well as social class and gender. Whereas the parents of a disturbed young woman in late nineteenth-century rural southwestern Japan might assume she was afflicted by a fox spirit, an urban middle-class husband witnessing his wife's spells of frenzied tearfulness a few decades later might wonder if she had developed a nervous illness. Over the course of the early twentieth century, families would increasingly participate in a commercialized economy of care, taking advantage of such new facilities as psychiatric hospitals, rest homes, and clinics. But many of these places either replicated or relied upon common idealizations of the gendered intimacies and hierarchies of familial relations in the provision of care, with male psychiatrists assuming the role of an all-knowing father-like figure and mostly female nurses tending to the everyday tasks of bodily and emotional care. Kin also wielded significant influence over the duration and nature of the treatments administered in places like psychiatric hospitals, to the extent that they could be seen as extensions of—rather than replacements for—domestic care.[2]

Although psychiatrists and some government officials tried to undermine long-standing family- and village-based structures of care, the passage of new legislation in the late nineteenth century ensured the continued primacy of familial responsibility for those considered mad. As part of its efforts to build the legal, political, and financial infrastructure necessary to resist Euro-American imperialist threats, the new Meiji government deployed a nationwide system of family registers in the early 1870s, which recorded every individual in the country as a member of a household under the control of a "household head," regardless of where the person lived. The Civil Code of 1898 then legally required households to support their destitute or ailing members, "establish[ing] an elaborate hierarchy of relationships that obligated the spouse, children and grandchildren, parents and grandparents, and then in-laws and siblings, reaching down to fairly distant relatives."[3] The Custody Law for the Mentally Ill of 1900 further enforced familial responsibility by requiring that all mentally disturbed individuals confined either at home or elsewhere have a designated legal custodian, ideally the male household head, who assumed legal responsibility. Meiji lawmakers and officials harnessed the power of existing practices of domestic responsibility to assert the family as the provider of care and relief for the needy and the linchpin of social order, thereby avoiding the costs of a state-funded welfare system.

Yet the family that mediated between afflicted members and institutions of law, medicine, and the state in the provision of care was not a stable and predetermined set of relationships defined exclusively by law, biology, or blood. The physical, mental, and financial demands of caregiving for those considered mad exposed family ties as fragile and contingent, created and tested in acts of everyday labor. The labor of care involved a range of activities, from filing paperwork with the proper authorities and hiring religious specialists to cleaning home confinement rooms. A disproportionate amount of this physical and mental labor fell on women, whether in rural farm households or middle-class families in cities. Women's bodies and minds performed much of the labor that helped constitute families, but this work was rendered invisible and uncompensated as a result of normative gender roles in the family. Such family-sustaining labor had its limits, too. Overworked and exhausted women and families were at times forced to relinquish care. Or, when mentally unstable individuals committed violent crimes, the state could not rely on families to manage them at home, as custom had dictated in preceding centuries, because new criminal laws held individuals, not families, responsible for crime.

When women were the ones to fall mentally, emotionally, or spiritually ill, family served as a crucial set of relationships through which they understood their experiences of illness. While their families and doctors located the source of affliction in their physiology and reproductive (mal)functions, many women narrated their experiences of illness by invoking the relations and language of kinship. In letters written to psychotherapists running rest homes, answers to questions asked by psychiatrists inside mental hospitals, and testimonies about their motivations to commit a crime, women repeatedly spoke of relations and obligations of family and local community—cheating husbands, slanderous neighbors, marriage possibilities, and more—in making sense of their illnesses and crimes. For them, their mental and emotional afflictions occurred not only within their bodies but in the realm of intimate social and familial relations. Their narratives of illness complicated those offered by their own families, as well as by psychiatrists and popular discourse.

The centrality of family in the care of those considered mad and in the creation of gendered understandings of madness is the subject of this book. The following chapters explain how the caregiving obligations of families intensified around the turn of the twentieth century, even as psychiatric ideas and institutions spread. Without the social welfare or medical policies necessary to make psychiatry accessible to the broader public, the burden of care continued to fall on families, especially the women therein. At the same time, this book shows how the gendered dynamics of family life produced vernacular understandings of kinship and madness that did not always conform to those promoted by the state or medical institutions. Rather than rely on legal formulations of the family or psychiatric explanations for mental afflictions, women turned instead to their own experiences of the intimate relations of kinship and community to make sense of their illnesses. As women and families navigated an unprecedented and shifting medical, legal, and commercial therapeutic landscape in turn-of-the-twentieth-century Japan, they produced a distinct set of gendered ideas and practices concerning care, bodies, and illness that would profoundly influence the everyday management of madness throughout the twentieth century and beyond.

Positioning Psychiatry

Focusing on the everyday experiences of women and families coping with madness allows for a re-evaluation of the impact of psychiatry in turn-of-the-twentieth-century Japan. Most studies of madness during this period, whether about Japan or another society, feature psychiatry and its institutions. This is not surprising, given that the nineteenth century witnessed the global rise of psychiatry as a medical science and profession, first in Europe and the United States and then in colonized or nearly colonized societies around the world.[4] Once an occasional pursuit, the study of madness became the full-time occupation of specialist physicians who began overseeing a range of institutions, from university departments to therapeutic asylums and private clinics. Confinement and treatment in such psychiatric institutions increased rapidly in many places, with numbers of asylum patients in Great Britain and the United States exploding from a few hundred to tens of thousands between the early 1800s and the early 1900s.[5] European colonies as far-flung as Algeria, India, and Singapore, as well as Japanese colonies such as Korea and Manchuria, saw the establishment of colonial asylums modeled on those in the metropoles: psychiatric ideas about racialized forms of madness developed there helped justify and sustain colonial rule.[6] Even as historians generally agree that asylums around the world failed to become the curative institutions that early psychiatrists had envisioned and that the source and extent of psychiatric influence varied across societies, they continue to focus on explaining the reasons for the expansion of psychiatric influence. Whether the result of support from new centralizing states, powerful new formulations of the normal and abnormal, or the collusion of such local actors as family and community, the centrality of psychiatry to studies of madness from the nineteenth century on is rarely questioned.

Scholars of madness in Japan have similarly been influenced by the fact that psychiatry was the newest and most publicized feature of the therapeutic landscape of madness at the turn of the twentieth century. Unlike in many formal European colonies where psychiatry and its institutions were often imposed on colonized peoples, Japanese officials, bureaucrats, and doctors actively chose to begin training medical students in German and Austrian psychiatry in the 1880s. Rejecting prevailing medical and religious explanations for madness such as spirit possession or blockages of bodily energy, the first Japanese psychiatrists introduced a biomedical model of mental disease through the new term *seishinbyō*. The literal translation of *seishinbyō*, "sickness of spirit," can be misleading because of its invocation of "spirit." But Japanese psychiatrists created the term to refer to biomedical diseases triggered by physical lesions in the brain, inherited psychological traits, or both.[7] Although the term is usually translated as "mental illness," it did not have the colloquial connotations that "mental illness" acquired elsewhere in the twentieth century. Instead, it remained a specialist term associated with severe mental diseases caused by biological—or what today would be called biochemical—malfunctions, which is the reason that neither the original term (*seishinbyō*) nor its English translation (mental illness) is used as a generic term for madness in this book. The psychiatrists claimed that such mental diseases required medical treatment in specialized institutions like the asylum or mental hospital rather than confinement and treatment at home, as had been common practice. Advertising their new ideas and facilities through public lectures, newspaper articles, and advertisements, psychiatrists aimed to debunk older beliefs and replace family-based management of madness with medical attention in psychiatric facilities.

These early psychiatrists seemed poised for success, especially since their efforts were supported by a new and ambitious government intent on integrating the nation—and later the Japanese empire—into the so-called modern world of science and medicine. Like many others globally, Japanese doctors and officials adopted European-influenced psychiatry in the 1870s in the context of Western imperialist threats. Two decades earlier, Japan had been forced to sign unequal treaties with the United States, France, Britain, Germany, and others under the pretense that the country was not "civilized" enough to maintain sovereignty. The provisions of the treaty marked Japan as a subjugated nation, unable to set its own import or export tariffs or adjudicate the crimes of Westerners in Japan. In the wake of a civil war in 1868 that toppled the previous military regime, the new Meiji government set out to demonstrate the nation's capacity for "civilization," understood in part as the ability to use the latest scientific and social knowledge in global circulation for the sake of national progress and power.

Among many other sweeping institutional changes, government officials and doctors began to build medical schools and institute a system of state licensing that legally elevated Western-derived medicine over older forms of medical practice.[8] After much debate, they chose German medicine as their model, hiring German physicians to teach in new state-sponsored medical schools.[9] Psychiatry soon became a part of the new curriculum, with Erwin Baelz in 1879 becoming the first physician hired to give lectures on psychiatry at what would later become Tokyo Imperial University. The government encouraged medical students to study psychiatry in Germany and Austria, too. In 1883, the Ministry of Education dispatched Sakaki Hajime, a recent medical school graduate, to study psychiatry in Berlin and tour state-supported asylums in Europe. Upon returning in 1887, Sakaki was named the first chair in psychiatric medicine at Tokyo University Medical School and the founding director of the Tokyo Public Asylum. Sakaki and the others who followed were elite Meiji men who hailed from prominent families of bureaucrats and physicians and were dedicated to leading the new Western-derived profession entrusted with helping to transform the country from "backward" to "civilized." From the 1910s to early 1940s, the students and successors of these early psychiatrists would extend their "civilizing mission" to such Japanese colonies as Korea and Manchuria.[10]

Yet the impact of psychiatry in Japan is difficult to assess. On the one hand, it introduced unprecedented ways of understanding and treating madness. As institutional histories have shown, hospitals as well as mental asylums were radically new spaces of care, with no precedents in Japan.[11] Some scholars have argued that psychiatry, in collusion with the state, acted as a repressive force in Japanese society, providing the language and justifications by which socially disruptive individuals and unorthodox religious groups were policed, incriminated, and controlled.[12] Others have shown the mechanisms of mass media and popular culture by which academic psychiatry and popular discourses on abnormality, deviance, and crime conditioned one another to create shifts, or "trends," in popular consciousness about mental and emotional affliction.[13] Psychiatry found platforms for its ideas in the military, law, criminology, sexology, and popular culture across the Japanese empire.[14]

Still, it remained a marginalized form of knowledge and practice. Psychiatrists struggled to change actual practices or treatments for madness on the ground, and campaigns to eliminate older beliefs about madness achieved limited success. Notions of psychological health rooted in older cosmologies of *ki* energy flowing in and throughout the mind and body persisted in everyday language. People continued to call upon religious healers for their unknowable ailments. And asylums and mental hospitals did not replace the home as the most common place of treatment. The number of such psychiatric institutions remained extremely limited. In 1918, the whole country had only one public asylum that housed about 450 patients and 57 private mental hospitals across the country treating about 4,000 patients.[15] Such facilities were limited to urban areas and even most city dwellers could not afford to pay the high admission and treatment fees. Psychiatric treatment remained associated only with the severest forms of madness.

Public awareness campaigns about mental hygiene, too, were short-lived. Many psychiatric ideas and concepts entered the public imagination and popular conversation, endowing the discipline with symbolic power as the most cutting-edge, scientific approach to madness, but this did not mean that the afflicted and their families were convinced that it would provide the best and most appropriate care. Japanese psychiatrists hardly achieved the status of their American or European counterparts who witnessed the rise of a "psychiatric persuasion," to use one historian's phrase, to assess the many aspects of everyday life, from eating habits to marital relations.[16] Psychiatry in turn-of-the-twentieth-century Japan generated a new language of madness, but failed to become the dominant institution to exert authority over madness.

One of the reasons Japanese psychiatry did not achieve hegemonic influence was that state officials and psychiatrists offered conflicting visions regarding the social and medical management of madness. The early Meiji government certainly supported the rise of elite men of medicine by employing them in such prestigious government-sponsored institutions as imperial universities and hospitals. It also backed psychiatric campaigns to redefine the phenomena of "fox attachment" as mental illness. But as early as the 1880s, it became clear that the state was more interested in the control of socially disruptive individuals and less concerned with healing or treating their conditions. Some of the first police ordinances in Tokyo concerning the removal off the streets and confinement in the new public asylum of those considered mad were motivated by the desire to remove unsightly people from city streets. Cleaning the cityscape in the aftermath of civil war was part of a larger project of so-called purification intended to impress foreign visitors or to make the streets traversable for the Meiji emperor. Once confined, whether in a poor house or by family, the mentally and spiritually disturbed individual was of less interest to the state. By contrast, psychiatrists considered themselves men of medicine who were invested in researching madness as a disease and curing those considered mad. Throughout the early twentieth century, they called repeatedly for the building of more public psychiatric hospitals. They succeeded in passing the Hospital Law of 1919, which required all prefectures to build at least one public asylum, but the state was not willing to meet the demands of the psychiatrists because it had found another means of ensuring that mentally disturbed individuals were properly managed: by reinforcing the responsibilities of the long-standing institution of the family.

Indeed, the family played a major role in managing madness in Japan, as seen in studies that have illuminated a variegated landscape of therapeutic care for those considered mad at the turn of the twentieth century. This landscape was characterized by a mix of formal medical care and informal domestic or local community-based care. Those in rural areas who used home confinement often sent their afflicted member to hospitals for temporary stays, alternating between domestic caging and psychiatric treatment. Others frequented what psychiatrists in official health inspection surveys at the time called "non-medical institutions," places such as "temples and shrines, waterfalls, hot springs, and others."[17] Often referred to as religious or folk therapies by scholars, they were few in number and scattered across the country, but their existence alongside psychiatric institutions further confirms the medical pluralism that characterized Japanese society at this time.[18] In fact, a number of psychiatric facilities were established near temples and shrines long associated with the care of those considered mad; an area known as Iwakura in northeast Kyoto was one of the most famous.[19] Both are examples of what historian Susan Burns has called "hybrid institutions," places with some medical oversight or historical associations with the past that helped publicize or sell their services.[20] A common but heretofore unacknowledged thread runs between these sites of care: all demanded the involvement of family. Fathers accompanied mentally disturbed sons to temples that offered such therapies as standing under a waterfall and incanting mantras. Mothers-in-law sent their daughters-in-law to medical clinics to receive treatment for nervous illnesses. Wives submitted petitions to local officials and police to build cages in which to confine their husbands. No matter the form of care, the presence of family was nearly universal.[21]

Histories of psychiatry concerning places other than Japan in the nineteenth and twentieth centuries have begun recasting families as active participants in the management of madness. Although most of these histories focus on North America and Western Europe, a cluster of recent works on colonial or semi-colonial societies such as India, Vietnam, and China have further shown the extent to which families around the world were not simply subjected to new psychiatric measures and institutions, but instead asserted some measure of control over the timing and terms of confinement and release, whether from an asylum, prison, or home.[22] The studies emphasize how families and ordinary people "used" such colonial institutions for their own ends, which rendered psychiatry's power diffuse and localized, rather than concentrated in hegemonic institutions of state and medicine.[23] Families are depicted as not necessarily resisting the state and psychiatric power, but "manipulating it to their own benefit."[24]

While recognizing that psychiatric power was constituted and contested with input from families, this book delves into the everyday experiences of families without using psychiatry as its main analytical framework. It aims to understand families' experiences on their own terms, discussing the role of psychiatry as one among many sources of institutional, practical, and moral claims with which families grappled when faced with decisions about diagnosis and care. Families encountered the claims of psychiatry and the state in a temporary and ad-hoc fashion. For instance, residents of rural villages in southwestern Japan briefly met Tokyo-based psychiatrists interested in recording cases of fox attachment in the 1880s and 1890s, but the encounter did not lead to a gradual erosion of long-standing cosmologies of animal spirits and madness. While national and prefectural laws concerning home confinement that specified details down to the mandatory size of padlocks on cage doors might give the impression that the custom came under sustained state surveillance, this was not the case in practice. Once the laborious process of applying for permission to confine was completed, most families were left on their own, for better or worse.

Nor did many families make decisions about confinement, treatment, or release based on whether they were manipulating—or being manipulated by—laws, government officials, or doctors. Instead they were driven by concerns like the allocation of limited resources such as money and labor as well as by long-standing ideas and expectations concerning the possibility of rehabilitating the mentally afflicted. They turned just as frequently to local religio-medical healers as they did to doctors trained in Western medicine. Those living in rural areas with no hospitals nearby often chose to confine mentally disturbed members prone to violence because no hand could be spared from the fields to watch over a troubled member. Families desperate to find cures for their afflicted member tried one treatment after another, whether at a Buddhist temple or psychiatric hospital. Even when families' decisions momentarily aligned with state interests, as in the desire of both to contain socially disruptive behavior, important differences existed. Families may have simultaneously hoped to rehabilitate their troublesome member, whereas the state was mostly interested in control and containment. By centering the experiences of families, and especially the women therein, it becomes possible to see how the intricacies of intimate and domestic life often determined the extent to which the claims and demands of various institutions of state, medicine, religion, and law gained traction.

Women and Families at the Center

Since at least the Edo period, the home had been the most common place of diagnosis and treatment of all illnesses, whether physical, mental, or both.[25] Daily contact meant that someone in the family, village, or neighborhood was most often the first to notice disturbing changes in a member's behavior or state of mind, from wandering aimlessly in the woods and babbling nonsense to inexplicably inflicting harm on themselves or others. If the strange and sometimes illegal behavior persisted or seemed to occur without good reason, families tended to suspect a case of madness. They often summoned a range of healers to their homes, including people who might be called religious and ritual therapists, but who were often referred to as "doctors" at the time—Buddhist priests, mountain ascetics, and itinerant priests. Elite and village-level practitioners of Sino-Japanese medicine made house calls, too, recommending herbal medicine and other remedies. Well into the twentieth century, a diverse array of healers and interveners converged on the space of the home, with families managing their comings and goings, as well as assessing their suggested remedies.

Despite criticism from the first Japanese psychiatrists and some sectors of the new Meiji state, the role of the family and its home in managing those considered mad, sick, or otherwise incapacitated was further institutionalized through law and ideology from the 1870s onward. Families had long been held responsible for their vulnerable members. Edo-period rulers had assigned the most immediate responsibility for poor relief to kin and local communities such as villages and neighborhood block associations, as well as often holding the same groups liable for crimes committed by individual members.[26] Yet the boundary between "family" and "community" had been ambiguous until the late nineteenth century, with other such communal units as "five-family groups" created for the purposes of paying taxes and assisting neighbors able to intervene in the management of members. Nor did families always want to care for impoverished or incapacitated relatives, especially when kinship ties were dubious or they had left their native villages.[27] Meiji leaders clarified and hardened this boundary through legislation. From the 1870s onward, Meiji laws began requiring every individual to be registered as a member of a unit known as the *ie* ("household" or "family") and remain under the control of a "household head" (*koshu*).[28] This new family registration system (*koseki*) ensured that every individual was officially affiliated with a household so that the state could hold the latter responsible for the welfare of their relatives.[29]

Within a few decades, the *ie* became a normative model of family enforced through the Civil Code of 1898, which then influenced new regulations concerning those considered mad.[30] As outlined in the Civil Code, the *ie* was organized as a hierarchy based on gender and seniority. In it a senior married couple lived with their eldest son and his wife and children. Either the senior male or the eldest son was designated as the male successor, who continued the family line by exercising nearly absolute power over subordinate members such as his wife, children, and younger males in the group. He alone managed the family property, determined the disposition of family assets, chose the family's place of residence, and approved or disallowed marriages and adoptions of his children. Building on ideologies and laws about the *ie* as outlined in the Civil Code, the first nationwide legislation concerning the management of the mentally ill in 1900 required all families to designate a "legal custodian" for any mentally disturbed member. Ideally the male household head, the legal custodian assumed legal and financial responsibility for the disturbed person. Whereas in the preceding era the "family" in charge of sick or otherwise incapacitated members could include a number of related and unrelated kin, Meiji laws required assigning responsibility to a single individual within an *ie*.

Male household heads may have ideally served as mentally afflicted individuals' legal custodians under the terms of the Custody Law of 1900, but it was mostly women who performed the daily physical and emotional labor of care. Women's caregiving labor was a crucial condition that made home-based care and confinement possible in the first place. Women's labor was essential for rural families living with home confinement, where women performed domestic chores for the confined, including laundering soiled bedding, preparing and delivering food, and cleaning makeshift toilets. For urban families, too, where a member might be hospitalized or coping with mental affliction at home, a disproportionate amount of caregiving was performed by women in the household, whether wives, mothers, daughters, or female servants. When women themselves became mentally and emotionally disturbed, they often tended to their conditions alone, turning to self-medication or consulting health manuals, magazines, and home encyclopedias, or in consultation with other women in their family, who might accompany them to visits with doctors or other healers.

The disproportionate burden of care placed on women was certainly not new in the Meiji period. Women from nearly all social classes in the preceding Edo period would have been expected to perform at least some of the physical labor of caring for the sick, which usually included cleaning bedding, administering medicines, receiving physicians and other healers, recording symptoms, helping with toilet needs, and cooking nourishing food. This was seen in popular fiction, didactic texts, diaries, and family records from the early nineteenth century. Although men, too, were often involved in sick-nursing, they were more likely to oversee decisions regarding the hiring of healers or to manage the movement of female relatives traveling from afar to assist with nursing.[31] The labor involved in caring for a mentally and spiritually afflicted member would have most likely been similar, since the distinction between mental and physical illnesses was not rigid in a medical and popular culture that understood bodily ailments in terms of the movement and stagnation of *ki* energy. Some differences existed, though. Attending to a mentally unstable member at times required more hands, especially if the person had to be physically restrained during bathing or toileting. Still, it is likely that the bulk of everyday care work fell on women, whether daughters-in-law, wives, or female servants, as it would in the decades that followed.

Women's household work acquired new meanings from the late nineteenth century onward as a gendered division of such labor became the cultural and social standard across classes. Before then, it was not unusual for men in commoner families to engage in cooking, housekeeping, and even childrearing. Women and men shared in such activities because all members of a family understood that the overarching goal was household continuity, not the well-being of individual members. So women and men, adults and children, and young and elderly alike partook in the work of perpetuating the family lineage, name, and occupation. Peasant mothers in poor and middling farming households, which constituted about 80 percent of the population, spent more time cultivating fields and silk reeling than toiling at domestic tasks like cooking and cleaning. Among these increasing numbers of entrepreneurial households, there was a less rigid distinction between women's and men's work, since the productive work of agriculture, handicrafts, sales, and customer service as well as the reproductive work of childrearing, shopping, cleaning, and cooking all took place at home. "The proximity of production and reproduction," argues historian Kathleen Uno, "allowed men, women, and children alike to participate in tasks crucial to the household's survival."[32]

In the late nineteenth century, expectations about household labor changed so that even as women, especially those in farm families, continued to perform productive work, men were no longer as involved in reproductive labor at home. Domestic work was increasingly gendered female as a result of the widespread influence of emergent structures and ideologies about a new middle- and upper-class model of womanhood and family. As Uno explains, "the destruction of old trades, the expansion of wage labor, and the rise of salaried workers created large-scale organizations like offices, government bureaus, and factories," which increasingly broke up production and reproduction tasks that had been carried out by households.[33] Men began to leave the home on a daily basis, especially in urban areas, as did children who were required to attend school for at least four years.

With the separation of school and workplace from the home, state officials, educators, social reformers, and others attempted to reshape women's roles so as to fit a new gender ideology often described by the slogan "good wife, wise mother."[34] Promoted by the Ministry of Education in 1898 and debated by educators, intellectuals, feminists, and young women, the slogan encapsulated the new expectation that young women would strive to achieve a domestic ideal rather than wage employment or political activities. Of course, the slogan was more official ideology than lived reality. Women from rural farm households and the urban poor never stopped working "outside" the home, and increasing numbers of middle-class women joined the workforce throughout the early twentieth century.[35] Still, "good wife, wise mother" became elevated as a social and cultural ideal across socioeconomic groups, raising the question of how a middle-class population of 6–8 percent of the country could set a norm that became the ideal for the other 90 percent or so.[36] But women's domestic activities were not consequently defined as "private" versus the labor of men in the workplace as "public," as one might expect. Instead, women's domestic work, embodied in the new figure of the "housewife" (*shufu*), was pursued as if it were a profession unto itself and as a service to state and nation that relied on the domestic expertise of women to enable the work of men and transform their children into good citizen–subjects.

These structural and ideological changes regarding the gendered division of household labor increased the actual importance of women's physical and affective labor in the maintenance of family life, but this labor has been rendered invisible by both contemporaries and historians. "Too ordinary or too unremarkable to be recorded in writing," as historian Mary Fissell has written about women's care work in early modern Europe, the "massive amounts of care" performed by women in Japan, too, rarely captured the attention of contemporary observers such as policemen collecting information about cases of home confinement or doctors and nurses watching family members tend to their relatives in mental hospitals.[37] Terms used to describe the everyday management of those considered mad that appear in medical and state archives also obscured the everyday physical and emotional labor of looking after an afflicted person. Government officials, police, and lawmakers concerned about minimizing social order used phrases such as "supervision and protection" (*kango*) and "confinement" (*kanchi*), while psychiatrists and other doctors deployed the language of "therapy" (*chiryō*) and "medical treatment." Such terms emphasized the bureaucratic surveillance and medical systems involved in managing madness, rather than the daily intensive work performed mostly by women.

Domestic care work has been underrepresented in histories of women's labor in turn-of-the-twentieth-century Japan. Most studies have focused on new forms of compensated labor that took place outside the home in factories, coal mines, cafes, retail venues, and schools.[38] Analyses of women's care work similarly tend to be limited to that which took place in new medical institutions such as hospitals by professional nurses and midwives.[39] When the domestic activities of women are the center of analyses, historians have rarely framed the childrearing, cooking, cleaning, or financial planning involved in "housewifery" as forms of care work.[40] But as recent studies of female maids in early twentieth-century Japan and its empire suggest, both housewives and female servants performed an immense amount of physical and emotional caregiving labor, whether in tending to sick or elderly relatives or maintaining "household harmony."[41] Framing the history of domestic labor as care work sheds light on the overlap between women's paid employment and unpaid domestic work, as well as the gendered nature and norms of care within familial settings.[42]

As cases of family-based management of madness reveal, the caregiving labor of women in turn-of-the-twentieth-century Japan consisted of mental, emotional, physical, and moral work that troubles common understandings of care. Care is often considered a universal and timeless virtue, a mode of engaging with others and responding to their needs in ways that create "the emotional foundations for solidarity" within communities.[43] It tends to be associated with "either good intentions, positive outcomes, or sentimental responses to suffering."[44] But care can also involve violence, repulsion, death, and ambivalent desires. Care does not always sustain or affirm life; it can prove lethal both to its recipients and givers, and it can take the form of allowing certain people to die.[45] In other words, care cannot be purged of its ambivalences. Such ambiguities are not readily captured by the terms and categories used by institutions of medicine, state, and law in turn-of-the-twentieth-century Japan.

Consider the evaluative terms deployed by psychiatrists to describe the material and hygienic conditions of cases of home confinement: good, ordinary, bad, and extremely bad. When the psychiatrists saw that the confined person was fed three times a day and taken out for walks regularly, they designated the case as "good." In cases where the confined were physically abused or their clothing and rooms left uncleaned, the psychiatrists condemned them as "bad" and "extremely bad."[46] Yet such evaluative terms made little sense when considered from the perspective of the family members performing the physical and emotional labor. As anthropologist Sarah Pinto suggests in her study of mental illness among women in contemporary India, such categories of ethical evaluation as good and bad, or care and abandonment, break down in the context of intimate relations: "In committing a family member to inpatient care, or managing a loved one's medication, or bringing a family member 'home,' or making a new home for oneself when things have come undone, care became—necessarily—indistinguishable from constraint; freedom felt a bit like abandonment."[47] It is likely that building a cage in which to confine one's husband or bringing a disturbed sister-in-law back home from a month-long stay at a private psychiatric hospital felt similarly fraught with contradiction. Was confining a family member in a wooden cage built inside the house a form of care or neglect? Was releasing a son from the demands of labor in the fields to spend a week in a temple receiving waterfall therapy as two strongmen held him down a form of freedom or abuse? These stark and often dichotomous categories of judgment broke down in the face of everyday and intimate experiences. Women and families usually inhabited gray zones of experience where a clear evaluation of the condition of care for the afflicted person might be nearly impossible, and any ensuing action or decision by family members was fraught with ambiguities, contradictions, and tensions.

Women's caregiving labor also upended the prevailing logic about the relationship between care and kinship. According to the laws, ideologies, and social norms of family obligation in turn-of-the-twentieth-century Japan, one supposedly cared for sick relatives because they were kin. The caregivers in this book show that the reverse happened, too: in providing care for a person, they created and confirmed kinship ties.[48] The labor of preparing food, washing bedding, summoning healers, and administering medicine enacted kinship in everyday life. In other words, kinship was not simply determined by blood, biology, or law, but could be constituted and validated through acts of labor.[49] Indeed, the labor of caregiving was sometimes performed by those "outside" the biological and legal kin group. Neighbors, servants, local officials, and even the state served as substitutes for family at times, making the boundary between family and non-family much more porous than one might expect. In refusing or becoming unable to provide care, one could weaken or dissolve kinship ties as well. The demands of managing madness involved a constant process of confirming but also questioning what exactly bound people as "family."[50]

Women's Afflictions in a Family Vernacular

As much as gender made family—that is, the disproportionate burden of daily caregiving labor placed on women enabled the intensification of the family-based care called for by the state—family made gender, too. Family life, in other words, reinforced the notion that experiences of mental disorder were differentiated by a gender binary of female and male. It did so by providing women a resource for creating a "family vernacular," or a gendered language that emphasized the interconnected nature of those within a kin network. After all, the family was one of the most immediate and officially sanctioned set of social and affective relations in which norms of gendered behavior were created, tested, and negotiated in everyday life. Families' initial diagnoses of a member's behavior as strange or abnormal and the subsequent decision on a course of treatment, too, was informed by assumptions about gender. As historian Akihito Suzuki has suggested in his study of the dispropor-tionate number of men in early twentieth-century Japanese mental asylums, the decisions of families to send their afflicted member to a psychiatric in-stitution or keep him or her at home hinged on gendered perceptions of an individual's level of "dangerousness."[51] Perceiving men as more prone to such serious acts of violence as murder and theft that affected strangers and others, families were more likely to send them to mental asylums while safeguarding afflicted women at home. The women, too, were seen as behaving in ways that were "dangerous" but more likely directed toward themselves in the form of suicide, disorderly conduct, and vagrancy than against others.

Of course, families did not adopt norms of gendered behavior in a cul-tural and social vacuum. At the turn of the twentieth century, families were compelled to navigate an increasingly complex array of popular and profes-sional discourses concerning gendered mental and emotional pathologies circulating in a range of media. Whether in newspapers, novels, short stories, advertisements, magazines, or exhibitions, one dominant interpre-tation emerged: women's mental and emotional afflictions could allegedly be attributed to their bodies, sexuality, and reproductive functions, whereas men's ailments tended to stem from an excessive performance of manual, physical, and intellectual work. This binary gendered distinction can be seen in the case of ideas and practices associated with "nervous illness" (*shinkeibyō*), with women increasingly identified with "hysteria" (*hisuterii*) and men with "nerve fatigue" (*shinkei suijaku*), or neurasthenia, beginning in the late nineteenth century.[52] Whereas hysteria was associated with a theatrical and dramatic excess of emotion, as well as violent bodily fits and spasms, neurasthenia featured symptoms such as headaches, withdrawnness, and taciturnity that contributed to the image of a brooding masculinity embodied by businessmen and intellectuals. Such a strongly dualistic gendered identification was produced mostly in the popular mass media.[53] Early psychiatrists tended, in fact, to downplay the gendered distinction, providing evidence of occurrences of hysteria among men.[54] But within families, the gendered distinction was pronounced, with mothers complaining about their married daughters showing signs of *hisu*, the casual abbreviation for the condition, and men describing their wives, older sisters, and aunts as having hysterical personalities that made the women susceptible to depression, anxiety, and excitability.

Gendered understandings of mental affliction in turn-of-the-twentieth-century Japan participated in a global scientific discourse that pathologized women's mental states and linked them to reproduction. Formulated by new professionals such as psychiatrists, sexologists, jurists, and criminologists in the nineteenth and twentieth centuries, theories about women's pathologies strove to identify the physiological sources of so-called deviant and transgressive behaviors of women. Physicians around the world cast women as "the product and prisoner of [their] reproductive system." Few questioned the assumption that the uterus and ovaries controlled the bodies and behavior of women from puberty through menopause, "whereas men's reproductive systems exerted no parallel degree of control over man's body."[55] Psychiatrists and criminologists in such places as Argentina, Brazil, Great Britain, the United States, Japan, and South Africa drew on such discourses to explain the madness of women, whether in relatively benign forms of nervousness or much more severe and debilitating cases of hysteria and schizophrenia.[56]

In their quest to locate bodily and inborn sources of mental and emotional deviance that influenced behavior, psychiatrists targeted their studies on women, suggesting that, despite possible differences in class, age, and personal history, the suffering of women might be narrowed down to a handful of diseases related to their reproductive functions and/or sexuality. When

Japanese psychiatrists descended upon rural villages wracked by cases of fox attachment, for example, they diagnosed the men with an array of ailments, including paranoia, mania, alcoholism, cholera, and typhus, but diagnosed 70 percent of the women with hysteria.[57] As historians and anthropologists have shown, such claims about the pathological nature of women's emotions and reproductive functions legitimated new fields of knowledge like gynecology and the (male) medical supervision of women.[58]

At the same time, the notion that disorders of women's reproductive organs could cause pathological reactions in other parts of the mind and body had deep roots in preceding centuries in Japan and elsewhere.[59] It was not uncommon to see "female madness" as a specific category of affliction explained as a result of "irregular menstruation" in popular and specialist Sino-Japanese medical handbooks in the late eighteenth and early nineteenth centuries.[60] Beyond medical discourse, intellectuals, social reformers, and others perpetuated ideas about women's physical and mental inferiority to men. For instance, female genitalia had long been linked to laziness, lasciviousness, and dull-wittedness in Edo-period neo-Confucian discourse. Mental and emotional disorders like hysteria and menstrual psychosis in the early twentieth century were, to some extent, new formulations of these older prejudices against women, repackaging Edo rhetoric about the unreliability and emotional volatility of women in a language of psychological and social pathology.[61]

Women and families engaged with these discourses in ways that defy assumptions about them simply accepting professional and popular discourses. Their engagement enabled women in particular to fashion vernacular narratives and cultural scripts of their own. Such dynamism can be best understood by considering the commercial context in which women and men, as well as experts and laypeople, encountered one another. The early twentieth century witnessed a considerable expansion of the medical marketplace, created in part by an oversupply of doctors, midwives, and other medical professionals graduating from state-sponsored programs and schools. Doctors competed to attract patients to their offices, clinics, and hospitals, as evidenced by the explosion of print advertisements for health services in national newspapers and magazines. Doctors thus appealed to the interests of women in their reproductive and family health as much as the latter may have been swayed by their claims of expertise. Nor were doctors the only people vying for the attention of women in the medical marketplace. Drug manufacturers, self-stylized healers, religious specialists, counselors, and other entrepreneurs offered treatments that differentially targeted women and men.

In the context of a burgeoning medical marketplace that provided no clear hierarchy of authority in regard to the knowledge and treatment of mental afflictions, many women painstakingly searched for explanations for their mental and bodily conditions that made sense to them in the context of their social and emotional lives. Of course, it is common for patients and families both then and now to wield explanatory models of illness that contradict, oppose, or simply ignore those offered by medical practitioners. Such explanatory models consist of informal descriptions of illness experiences that are usually tacit, self-contradictory, and ever-shifting in content. They are, as anthropologist Arthur Kleinman suggests, "our representations of the cultural flow of life experience," and therefore "congeal and unravel as that flow and our understanding of it firms up in one situation only to dissolve in another."[62] This book traces the contours of the "cultural flow of life experience"—or the ideas about their bodies and illness that the women took for granted, or were so immersed within that they might not have been able to lift themselves out of the flow in order to observe.

One of the key features of this "cultural flow of life experience" that shaped women's understandings of their mental, emotional, and spiritual afflictions was the notion that their illnesses occurred "off" the body, to borrow the words of anthropologists Veena Das and Renu Addlakha, and in the realm of intimate, family relations.[63] Women often refused to localize their illnesses in their individual minds and bodies, invoking instead the influence of kin and family in the shaping of their suffering. Nonetheless, there were competing claims about whether an illness occurred "in" or "off" a particular body. While families and doctors in Japan were often interested in isolating the affliction within the body of the woman, the women themselves tended to point to the ways in which their bodies were inseparable from the world of family and kin, often the source of both crisis and comfort.

Still, women did not entirely discount the role of their bodies. But instead of invoking only the language of contemporary doctors and other specialists, women drew on an older and influential Sino-Japanese medical and cultural model of "flow," which saw blockages, stagnation, knotting, and congelation of psycho-spiritual forces like vital energy (*ki*) and blood as sources of sickness.[64] Invoking ideas about blood-flow reversals, the women produced their own interpretations of mental distress that resonated with but still questioned new biomedical notions of female pain. In doing so, they created their own vernacular vocabularies, narratives, and cultural scripts of female madness that persist to this day.

Sites of Encounter

Each of the following chapters explores a site of encounter—the rural village, farm household, urban marketplace, and courtroom—to trace the various ways in which family was central in the care of those considered mad as well as in the creation of gendered understandings of madness. The sites are both actual places and conceptual spaces where the claims and practices of women and families interfaced with those of the state, medicine, law, markets, and religion in turn-of-the-twentieth-century Japan. In each site, the characteristics of such institutions are not treated as "givens." Instead, the nature and effects of these institutions emerge in relation to one another and through the process of description.[65] The analysis in this book highlights how and where the institutions intersected or bypassed one another in the context of a specific site of encounter.

The book begins in the remote villages of southwestern Japan, famous for their cases of fox attachment. Chapter 1, "Fox Spirits in Villages," illuminates a crucial moment in Meiji history when newly organized groups of people, namely Meiji government officials and psychiatrists, attempted to establish their authority in ways that undermined preexisting family- and village-centered structures and cultures of religious and spiritual care for those considered mad. The home had long been the most common site of care and custody to which families summoned a range of medico-religious healers and others to tend to the physically, mentally, and spiritually sick. With the support of the new Meiji state, the first Japanese psychiatrists of the 1880s challenged the notion of fox attachment as well as family-centered care, redefining fox attachment as a sexualized "mental illness" that would be best treated within the walls of mental asylums.

Yet their efforts to redefine these ailments as "mental illness" had limited effects. Well into the late nineteenth and early twentieth centuries, fox attachment wielded power as a language and mode of filiation in the context of familial and village life. Cases of fox attachment showed how filiation, or ways in which one living being was put in relation to another, occurred along lines other than those of blood, biology, or law. As the parameters of the language of "attachment" expanded, it would bring into its purview some of the most tumultuous global and local phenomena of Meiji Japan, from conscription and cholera to treaty-port imperialism.

The persistence of family-based care for those considered mad becomes especially apparent in looking at home confinement, a practice by which those considered mad and prone to violence were confined in cage-like structures built inside the family home. Chapter 2, "Cages in Rural Homes," shows how family-based care intensified through the legal and bureaucratic institution-alization of familial responsibility for those considered mad or otherwise in-capacitated. More important, it analyzes a condition of possibility for home confinement that has long been rendered invisible: a domestic and moral economy of caregiving that heavily relied on women's physical and mental labor. Women mustered the energy to make life as livable as possible for the people with and for whom they felt intimate, indebted, or responsible by performing the bulk of the intensive labor of care, from cleaning bedding and toilets, to supervising hospital visits and administering medication. This gendered labor, taken for granted by observers, helped create the social and emotional ties by which the relations of family were rendered meaningful in everyday life. But just as readily, the demand and toll of the labor could attenuate ties of kinship and call into question what exactly was considered "normal" family relations.

Linked to rural areas where fox spirits were said to roam and women cared for confined family members were booming cities in which a burgeoning med-ical marketplace began targeting an increasing number of women diagnosed with hysteria, the subject of Chapter 3, "Hysteria in the Marketplace." Between the mid-1910s and early 1930s, drug manufacturers, medical professionals, self-stylized healers, religious specialists, and other entrepreneurs offered treatments for hysteria and other similar nervous conditions that extended sites of care from the home to an eclectic array of places, including private clinics, rest homes, religious centers, and even police-led personal con-sultation offices. Although such services became available to middle- and upper-class consumers leading a "life of therapy" (*ryōhō seikatsu*) in search of remedies for their sufferings, the diagnosis and search for treatments was still guided by "family" in two senses of the term. First, such family members as mothers, sisters, and husbands helped afflicted individuals navigate the med-ical marketplace. At the same time, afflicted women often identified these very families, as well as the tensions produced by the obligations and affective re-lations within them, as a source of their pain. Second, the women made sense of their afflictions by using a family vernacular, situating their illnesses within the intimate relations of family and kin, even as they sought cures in such therapeutic facilities as "rest homes" that replicated some of the structures of paternalistic family-based care.

Yet the reliance on family-based care had its limits. Chapter 4, "Periodic Crimes in the Courtroom," shows how cases of violent crime compelled families to relinquish responsibility, shifting care provision and management from the space of the home to that of the courtroom. Focusing on criminal cases of women who allegedly suffered from menstruation-induced mental instability at the time of their crimes in the 1920s and 1930s, this final chapter examines how the family could no longer function as the liable unit in cases of crime once new criminal laws from the 1870s to 1907 held individuals—and not families, as had been the case in the preceding Edo period—responsible for their unlawful activity. Individuation within the context of criminal law was a gendered process, for it involved differentiating between the gendered bodies of women and men, as seen in cases of menstruation-induced mental instability. In the context of a judicial process that aimed to individuate a female defendant's body as much as possible, the women themselves simultaneously bolstered notions of individual autonomy found in psychiatric and legal discourse and offered distinct understandings of their allegedly mad criminal acts as having emanated from embodied experiences within the domain of kinship. The courtroom, too, contained instances of women using the family vernacular—infused with an older language of "bloody inversion," or the experience of upheavals of nervous energies and blood flows—to make sense of the workings of their minds and bodies.

Finally, the Epilogue, "Postwar Cultures of Gendered Care and Kinship," considers the continuation of turn-of-the-twentieth-century gendered understandings of madness and family-based care into the post–World War II period and beyond. In the early 1950s, a series of laws and financial incentives dramatically shifted structures of care. For the first time, hospitals replaced the home as the most common site of treatment for severe mental illnesses. Still, families retained their primacy in the management of care to some extent. They made the initial decision to send relatives to psychiatric hospitals, served as a crucial node in a network of home- and hospital-based care, and worked as unpaid auxiliary caregivers within hospitals. Indeed, the burden of domestic responsibility for the mentally ill fell even more intensely on the shoulders of women than ever before, as the home was renewed as the most socially legitimate space of rest. Gendered notions of madness persisted, too, as did women's reliance on the language of kinship and domesticity to make sense of various forms of mental and emotional distress, many of which came in the guise of updated diagnostic categories. Women's various uses of these categories suggest that they continue to interpret their bodily and psychic health through the framework of kinship because no public narrative about the structural reasons for women's distresses exists.

To trace the movements of people, practices, and ideas within and between these sites of encounter, this book attends to what has been called the "rough ground of the ordinary."[66] The analysis looks to the ground on which families tread to follow their actual movements, noting their travels from one site of healing to another or from a rural household to an urban hospital and back, while still recognizing the immobility of some families, especially those with fewer resources of labor, money, and kin networks. It illuminates the bits and fragments of stories concerning an array of anonymous families who entered the historical record usually in the moments they encountered institutions of state and psychiatry. State- and psychiatric-produced documents can be read to reveal the ways in which they expose everyday details about the physical and emotional labor of women that created but also tested and attenuated ties of family. Seemingly mundane details recorded about a female defendant's menstrual cycle or a psychiatrist-ethnographer's description of a young woman afflicted by a fox spirit point to an uneven terrain of everyday life that exposes how such institutions as family and medicine functioned, or ceased to function, in relation to one another, whether through legal codification, cultural representations, female sociality, gendered labor, or vernacular expressions.

The book also follows the diverse and often-contradictory vocabularies and narratives of madness deployed by women and families. Such vocabularies and narratives were specific to a range of social geographies, from gender and location to social status and occupation. In the following pages, terms like "madness" and "mental affliction" serve as generic signifiers for mental and emotional conditions considered abnormal, strange, or otherwise inexplicable in their historical contexts. "Mental illness" appears in relevant contexts, especially where psychiatric discourse and categories are invoked, but not as the catch-all descriptor that it often is deployed as in medical and popular discourse today. In fact, women and families rarely used the term "mental illness," preferring instead the more general term "illness" (*byōki* or *yamai*) even to describe non-physiological ailments. They deployed more specific terms, too: "flare-ups," "hysteria," "fox attachment," "crazy," and "sick." Wherever possible, the generic and specific terms of women and families guide the analysis of this book, showing how they amplified but also countered terms deployed in psychiatric, legal, and criminological discourses.

Along with social geography, vocabularies of madness were shaped by the historical moments in which they were deployed. But time, when traced through shifts in vocabularies of madness, appears more disjointed than continuous, more fragmented than smooth, as older ideas can be passed down and intertwine with newer ones. Pasts inhabit presents and even futures.[67] People's lives and words occupy more than one temporality at a time, as so evocatively evidenced by the language of blood flow—its reversals, imbalances, and excesses—as it would trickle down through the centuries to enter the twentieth-century discourses of Japanese psychiatrists and women alike to explain the functioning of women's bodies and minds. Such languages and ways of living with madness infused with multiple temporalities, as well as the women and families who shaped the gendered nature of care and illness, become visible through alternating long and close-up shots of overlapping sites of encounter.

The following chapters thus present an episodic history of madness in the family, one that shows how experiences of madness, kinship, gender, and care were entangled with one another in different ways in a range of sites across turn-of-the-twentieth-century Japan. Treating individuals afflicted by fox spirits required confronting inter-family tensions within rural villages. Madness exposed forms of kinship along supernatural, communal, and matrilineal lines that did not fit normative visions of family. Kinship itself proved fragile when women faced the grueling demands of everyday care. In other instances, kinship ties became sources of both suffering and succor. After all, women were often compelled to rely on their kin networks for both an explanatory framework for their illnesses as well as everyday care. Such entanglements, in turn, render entities such as "the family" and "care" that so many, back then and now, might claim to know through study, intuition, or personal experience, into unfamiliar subjects of history.

Fox Spirits in Villages

IN 1882, IN the town of Kita-adachi in Saitama prefecture, a relatively well-to-do farmer named Kazayo Yūjirō discovered that all five members of his family had gone mad (*hakkyō shita*). His wife and children burst into uncontrollable fits of laughter one moment, only to fly into a rage the next, as if stricken by some unknown force. This is no small matter, thought Kazayo. If I don't get help, my family will be overcome by madness (*kichigai ni naru*). Believing that the cause might be a curse of the local protector deity, Kazayo rushed to the nearby shrine to seek advice from the priest. The priest consulted the gods and identified the cause of the strange behavior with uncanny precision: it was most certainly Tanaka Ichigorō, the leader of a rival religious group associated with Mt. Mitake, who had unleashed a fox spirit on the Kazayo family to bewitch them into a frenzy. The revelation infuriated not only Kazayo but also the young men of Kita-adachi. How dare this Ichigorō send a fox spirit to torment the people of their town! Wrapping towels around their foreheads and raising their hoes in the air, they shouted for Tanaka's head.

But before the violence escalated, an elder of Kita-adachi warned that the gods would not forgive an uprising and suggested instead that the men file a complaint with the police. The men put their accusation in writing and submitted a petition at the police headquarters in nearby Sōka. The police dismissed the petition with disdain, declaring that there was no such thing as fox spirits overtaking the minds and bodies of people and that the Kazayo family was simply ill. The Sōka police headquarters dispatched one of its men to find a doctor (*isha*) and accompany him to the Kazayo residence, where he treated the family and, lo and behold, cured them of their madness. Only then did the men of Kita-adachi take to heart the words of the police.[1]

At first glance, the story of Kazayo appears to affirm the stance of early Meiji leaders that commoners ought to be disabused of so-called superstitions

Madness in the Family. H. Yumi Kim, Oxford University Press. © Oxford University Press 2022.
DOI: 10.1093/oso/9780197507353.003.0002

that hampered efforts to "civilize and enlighten" the nation in the face of European and American imperialist aggression in the late nineteenth century. Reported in one of the first national newspapers, Kazayo's story involved a Meiji policeman and doctor persuading a group of farmers that madness originated not in fox spirits, but sickness. Meiji reformers blamed such allegedly wayward beliefs about fox spirits for causing unnecessary social upheaval, like the one nearly carried out by the men of Kita-adachi, and preventing Japan from gaining international recognition as a civilized nation worthy of equal treatment by Western powers. In the 1870s and 1880s, officials, intellectuals, doctors, and reformers waged an "anti-superstition campaign," circulating reports of the undesirable consequences of ideas and rituals related to animal spirits and exorcism.[2] Most contemporaries deemed the campaign successful by the early twentieth century. A newspaper headline in 1932 announced that "the figure of the fox spirit [that overtakes humans] has disappeared, and the number of mentally ill persons has escalated."[3] The alleged few who held fast to notions of shape-shifting foxes were labeled as superstitious and ignorant, stuck in a primitive world of unreason and unable to move forward with the times. With the introduction of a so-called scientific explanation, foxes were supposedly divested of their power to mediate between the human and spirit realms, the curtain falling on a time and space once charged with supernatural possibilities.

Yet the story of Kazayo might be read another way. In the course of lauding the police and doctor for supposedly shattering illusions about fox spirits, the reporter reveals the ways in which Kazayo faced an array of clashing claims about the cause of his family's strange behavior as well as the proper authorities with whom he ought to consult. Consider the competition among religious specialists. The local priest fuels intra-religious conflict by identifying a rival religious practitioner as the culprit responsible for unleashing foxes. Such rivalries may have originated in the preceding Edo period, but many were newly created by Meiji policies that pit religious groups against one another and forced many clerics and practitioners to forge new alliances or discontinue their activities. The policies originated in attempts by the fledgling Meiji state to legitimize the political coup that overthrew the previous military regime and restored imperial rule. Nor are the state-sponsored police and doctor the only sources of authority in the story. Other influential figures include the protector deity and the town elder, neither of whom fit neatly into the binary division between so-called modernizing elite and superstitious folk. In fact, the townsmen first turn to the police out of either respect or fear of not only the elder, but also the local deity who might unleash its wrath if the men launched an upheaval. To decide on a proper course of action, Kazayo and his fellow townsmen navigate the competing and overlapping claims of authorities old and new.

Kazayo's story belongs to a crucial moment in Meiji history when government officials and psychiatrists attempted to establish their authority in ways that undermined preexisting family- and village-centered structures and cultures of religious and spiritual care for those considered mad. Each group had its own reasons for launching an offense against practices associated with fox-spirit-induced madness. National government officials aimed to delegitimize local religious specialists whose ritual activities drew from cosmologies that had supported the political structures of the previous Tokugawa regime. Prefectural and other local government officials attempted to eliminate family-based practices related to fox spirits that they believed led to social disorder. Psychiatrists joined the government-led offense by offering such gendered and sexualized notions of madness as hysteria as an alternative explanation for the disturbed states of mind seen among those affected by foxes. Through publications of their clinical research in the nation's first asylums, lectures for civic associations, and ethnographic surveys of regions known for fox-spirit-induced madness, psychiatrists claimed that the only legitimate source of diagnosis and treatment for such cases was not the family, but medical theories and institutions.

Yet efforts to redefine fox-spirit-related ailments as "superstition" and "mental illness" had limited effects. Long into the late nineteenth and early twentieth centuries, "fox attachment" or "fox-spirit attachment" (*kitsune tsuki*) wielded power as a language and mode of filiation in the context of familial and village life. Although *kitsune tsuki* is commonly translated in English as "fox possession" or "fox-spirit possession," "attachment" is used here instead to retain the literal meaning of *tsuku*, the Japanese verb from which *tsuki* derives. This literal translation helps maintain the sense in the original Japanese of a spatial and tactile technique of adherence through which one entity comes into contact with another. *Tsuki* conjures a form of superficial contact, one that occurs at the surface, as if fox spirits and humans are two surfaces that stick to one another, rather than a deep and penetrating form of control and ownership, as the English word "possession" suggests. The translation of *tsuki* as "attachment" takes families on their own terms, both literally and figuratively. Tracing the evocative ways in which the language of "attachment" was enmeshed with that of family in late nineteenth-century Japan illuminates the existence of a provocative array of kinship forms that were increasingly bound together with but also outside the purview of the state.

Surface-level attachments produced various forms of filiation, or ways in which one living being was put in relation to another. Filiation that occurred through acts of *tsuki*, or attachment, could be temporary or much longer-lasting, passed down through the generations. When a fox spirit attached itself to an individual in the villages of southwestern Japan, the affected family assumed that another family had sent the spirit in malice. If a man married into one of these fox-wielding families, he and his descendants would be forever associated with fox spirits. Considering filiation through the language of *tsuki* thus provides a glimpse into a world in which there were possibilities beyond blood, biology, or the law to create, affirm, and weaken ties of kinship and community. When Meiji officials and psychiatrists entered this world of "attachment," their efforts to dismantle it sometimes further amplified its powers. Official and psychiatric records show the expansion of the parameters of the language of "attachment," one that helped make sense of some of the most tumultuous global and local phenomena of Meiji Japan, from conscription and cholera to treaty-port imperialism. Some of the new claims by state officials and psychiatrists certainly managed to stick in some contexts, but the ability of the world of "attachment" to continue to generate dynamic notions of filiation and kinship, especially in rural villages, proved powerful and persistent.

Family-based Management of Madness in the Edo Period

When the first Japanese psychiatrists descended upon rural villages known for their cases of fox attachment, they witnessed what would have been a familiar world even to their professional urbanite eyes: families—not doctors—managed the diagnosis and treatment of mental, emotional, and spiritual afflictions. Usually consisting of a group of kin and non-kin dependents such as servants and staff who lived all together, families had occupied a central role in managing illnesses of mind and body since at least the sixteenth century.[4] Daily contact meant that someone in the family was most often the first to notice disturbing changes in a member's behavior or state of mind, from wandering aimlessly in the woods and babbling nonsense to inexplicably self-harming or inflicting harm on others. If the strange and sometimes illegal behavior persisted or seemed to occur without good reason, families tended to suspect a case of madness.

Edo-period families speculated about the cause or nature of a member's madness, often with the input of fellow villagers and acquaintances. Most commonly, people used such terms as *kichigai* (気違い) and *ranki* (乱気)

for madness, invoking the widespread philosophical and medical notion of *ki*
(気), or "vital energy."[5] An invisible and intangible life force, *ki* constituted
the flow of energy that circulated both within the body and between the
body and the environment. During its circulation through and between living
things, *ki* could both change or be changed by a range of such social, affective,
material, or natural forces as interpersonal relations, emotions, or wind and
cold. *Ki* might surge in anger, drain away in sorrow, or become knotted when
exercising caution.[6] It was considered a significant determinant of health and
illness, with disruptions in its smooth flow seen as a potential cause of bodily
and psychological suffering. The term *kichigai* thus suggested that the flow
of *ki* had become "altered" or "different" and is still used today as a colloquial expression to describe strange behavior. Similarly, *ranki* described *ki*
as having been "disordered." Other analogous terms for madness included
ranshin ("disordered heart") and *jōki* ("elevated *ki*"), as recorded in Edo-
period documents composed by village headmen, city magistrates, and other
officials compelled to identify cases of madness when executing punishments
for crimes or granting permission for home confinement.[7]

Understandings of madness as caused by *ki* disturbances were reinforced
by a growing Sino-Japanese medical literature on the topic in the eighteenth
century. Japanese physicians trained in this "Chinese method" (*kanpō*) of
medicine increasingly identified the cause of psychological disorder in the
stagnation of *ki* in such organs of the body as the heart, stomach, or liver.[8]
Famous *kanpō* physicians such as Wada Tokaku proposed that blockages of
ki in the liver affected one's emotional and mental state. Wada theorized that
such moral failings as idleness, indolence, and indulgence could cause the
ki in the liver to "lose tension," which led to various mental and emotional
disorders.[9] Another related and widespread term deriving from Sino-Japanese
medicine was *kan*. Although *kan* was associated with convulsions and seizures
in the medical literature, it became popularized as the expression *kanshō*, literally meaning either "*kan* nature" (癇性) or "*kan* symptoms" (癇症), to
describe people who were anxious, fastidious, obsessed with cleanliness, or
pompous.[10] Since *kan* was also homonym for "liver," *kanshō* was at times
written as "liver symptoms" (肝症).[11] Even today the same term is widely used
to describe individuals with nervous and obsessive personalities, similar to the
way the psychiatric term "OCD" (obsessive-compulsive disorder) is used in
colloquial English to describe those who are excessively orderly.

Like *kanpō*-derived explanations of madness, fox attachment involved
ideas about the body as porous to elements in the surrounding environment, including "things that attached" (*tsukimono*). Along with deities and

ghosts of deceased persons, the spirits of such animals as foxes, "racoon-dogs" (*tanuki*), "dog-spirits" (*inugami*), cats, and snakes were said to "attach" to people, overtaking their minds and bodies.[12] The animal spirits were known for using humans as hosts in both mischievous and serious ways, whether playing pranks on innocent bystanders or exacting revenge.[13] So when families, neighbors, or even passersby heard that an afflicted person had asked for red-bean rice or tofu, foods thought to be favored by foxes, or recalled that the person had recently visited a shrine that worshipped Inari, a deity for which the shape-shifting fox was a symbol, they might guess that a fox spirit had "attached" itself to the person and triggered mad behavior.

Fox attachment was widely known as an explanation for madness, but was more frequently invoked in some parts of the country than in others. The rural areas of southwestern Japan that psychiatrists would visit in the late nineteenth century, for example, were well known for cases of fox attachment. Still, major urban areas like Edo or Kyoto as well as regions in the northeast reported cases, too. As historian Hiruta Genshirō has shown in his study of Moriyama domain in present-day Fukushima prefecture, some officials and families recorded instances of fox attachment in cases of unexpected suicides and murders that could not be explained otherwise.[14]

Whether families determined that their member suffering from madness was afflicted with a *ki*-related disorder, fox spirit, or something else, nearly all would have first turned to religious and ritual therapy provided by such healers as Buddhist priests, mountain ascetics (*yamabushi* or *Shugenja*), itinerant priests, and holy men (*hijiri*). This is perhaps not surprising in cases of fox attachment, which tends to be seen as a supernatural or magical phenomenon treated by religious healers who performed exorcisms. Religious specialists affiliated with esoteric sects like Shingon were especially famous for performing spirit exorcisms and related prayer rituals, while others deployed ritual tools like writing characters on special paper and attaching them to the bodies of the afflicted.[15]

Less known is how the same religious specialists served as the main providers of medicine and healing for most Japanese well into the nineteenth century, no matter the physical or spiritual ailment. Many Buddhist priests had been educated in medical studies since at least the medieval period.[16] Temples often sold their own proprietary herbal medicine, as did itinerant priests associated with famous holy sites, so much so that peddlers of medicine often dressed in priestly garb to signal their legitimacy and thereby attract more customers. Certain popular medicines were tied to the miraculous powers of Buddhist, Taoist, or Shinto deities as well.[17] So when families

summoned religious specialists to treat cases of fox attachment, they were
not rejecting the methods of medical doctors or physicians, but rather calling
upon healers who were among the most sought-out for medical care and
treatment. Religious healers were often even referred to as "doctors" (*i*).

The prevalence of religious and ritual therapy across social classes has
been obscured by a scholarly focus on the rise of "rational" schools of neo-
Confucian, nativist, and Western medical traditions.[18] It is true that such
traditions became more widely accessible to people beyond the urban social elite in the late eighteenth century. The numbers of local village doctors
influenced by elite practitioners, for instance, increased exponentially in
the countryside. Individuals named as "doctors" had rarely appeared in
seventeenth-century local records and diaries of village elites, but after 1750
the number of mentions of village-level physicians increased.[19] Some rural
families coping with madness certainly called on such doctors, who tended
to administer herbal medicine and emetics as treatment for cases of madness.
Still, these village doctors, along with their urban counterparts, did not replace religious specialists as the most commonly hired healers of illness. In
fact, doctors in cities, towns, and villages worked to distinguish themselves
as providers of "medical" care, as opposed to what they called magical and
ritual healing by religious specialists. The birth of such a distinction between
"medical" and "magical" or "religious" therapies in the late eighteenth century
originated in this competition in an expanding medical marketplace.

Indeed, Edo-period families sought out an array of healers and treatments
in a fluid and pluralistic way. With no institutionalized hierarchy of healers in
place, as there would be later in the Meiji period, people did not necessarily
grant a doctor trained in Sino-Japanese medicine (*kanpō*) with more legitimacy. Nor was there a rigid distinction between healers who treated spirit-
attachment-related ailments and those who tended to physical ones. Even
as many doctors distinguished themselves from so-called magico-religious
therapeutics, some still diagnosed and treated fox attachment. When *kanpō*
physician Nakagami Kinkei was hired by a family of a sixteen-year-old girl
who was waking up in the middle of the night and dancing until sunrise, he
agreed with her parents' assessment that a fox spirit had attached itself to
her, for which he prescribed herbal sedatives. In this case, as well as in others,
families readily hired one healer after another until they found an effective
treatment.[20]

Kanpō doctor Kitamura Ryōtaku was one among many healers hired by
a family of a woman who showed signs of madness after visiting a famous
Inari shrine at the edges of Edo city. She sung loudly, talked incoherently, and

claimed that she could read minds. Those around her believed that a fox spirit had attached itself to her, likely because she had visited an Inari shrine, which was associated with foxes. Kitamura made note of all the healers who had been summoned before him: a monk who chanted a sutra, a doctor (*i*) who tried to expel the fox spirit from her body by burning incense, a warrior who attempted to scare the fox spirit away with a bow and arrow, and a doctor who boiled "farewell money" (*senbetsu*) to persuade the fox to be on its way and then gave her the infusion to drink. Even Kitamura invoked common parlance, referring to the healers who burned incense and boiled farewell money as "doctors" (*i*), which at the time included what one might now conventionally call religious or spiritual healers.[21] The reference to the warrior also confirms that families did not exclusively turn to those who specialized in healing to treat fox-spirit attachment. Members of the warrior class (*bushi*), for instance, were summoned to frighten off fox spirits with their weapons. Indeed, families called upon neighbors, relatives, siblings, local officials, and others who had no special training but would try to persuade and reprimand the fox spirit to leave the afflicted person's body.[22]

A diverse array of healers and interveners converged on the space of the home, with families managing their comings and goings, as well as assessing their suggested remedies. As historian Evan Young has argued, "doctoring was a mobile profession, one practiced in the homes of patients" at a time when hospitals and clinics were nearly nonexistent.[23] Families did not rely on a single trusted physician, but instead tended to hire a series of different doctors and healers. Doctors often arrived well after the onset of symptoms and consultations with other healers. Their knowledge of the patient's illness, as well as any attempted treatments, was limited to what the family decided to divulge, and they spent relatively little time with their patients over the course of an illness. "[T]he home remained the center of therapy," writes Young, "and it was there where families cared for ailing loved ones, where they interacted with medical practitioners, and where they tried new medicines and observed firsthand whether the treatments had any effect."[24] With families wielding the most decision-making power and their homes serving as "the center of therapy," visiting doctors and other healers played more of a supplementary role.

Distinctions between types of healers would harden in the Meiji period. Although the medical marketplace would only become more competitive after 1868, a new state-supported medical system of licensing and an accompanying denigration of so-called traditional and folk therapies created an official hierarchy of healers with Western-trained doctors at the top and *kanpō* doctors below. Of course, the implementation of a new state-led medical system did not change the therapeutic landscape overnight. Options in terms of treatment and care provision remained constrained by the types of healers that were practically and financially accessible to families. Still, state officials and reformers began pursuing their own agendas of political and medical reform after 1868, trying to undermine structures and cultures of family-centered religious and medical care. The official and psychiatric attack on fox attachment constituted one such attempt.

State and Psychiatric Interventions

Meiji government officials, ideologues, and intellectuals waged war against fox spirits as part of a broader effort to legitimize the political coup that toppled the previous Tokugawa regime. Nativist scholars who supported the coup quickly put their scholarship to work in the interest of the new leaders. They provided a rhetoric of imperial restoration, denouncing the Tokugawa for having usurped imperial power and praising the coup leaders for restoring imperial rule. Like the first emperor of Japan in the seventh century, the Meiji emperor would rule according to the will of his divine ancestor, Amaterasu. Restoring the ancient purity of imperial rule, however, required a purge of the "foreign" beliefs, including the blending of local native gods (*kami*) within a larger Buddhist cosmology that had supported the political structures of the Tokugawa regime. To re-establish ancient purity, the government began to issue a series of edicts to "separate the kami from the buddhas." The edicts ordered the disassociation of the kami from the allegedly foreign buddhas derived from Indian and Chinese belief systems. The disassociation required a diverse group of religious specialists who had long combined ideas and practices from various traditions to choose to become either shrine priests or Buddhist clerics, with no option in between. It also elevated *kami* worship above Buddhism, leading to the state support of the former and persecution of the latter.[25]

The edicts singled out the activities of *yamabushi*, a group of religious specialists associated with the mountain-based tradition of Shugendō who deployed magic, exorcism, and ritual prayers as part of their ritual and healing services. In 1872, the Council of State (Dajōkan) banned Shugendō, forcing its practitioners to join Buddhist orders. Officials curtailed the kinds of rituals that had commonly sustained *yamabushi* as well as other such religious specialists as spirit mediums, oracles, fortune tellers, itinerants, and diviners. In 1873, the Ministry of Doctrine outlawed the various activities of "traditional

catalpa diviners [*azusamiko*], female mediums [*ichiko*], and those who practice spirit-possession rituals [*hyōkitō*], fox summoning [*kitsune sage*], coin div-
ination and spirit-speaking [*kuchiyose*]" because they allegedly "bedazzled"
(*genwaku*) the general populace, leading them astray and often swindling
them.²⁶ Prohibitions against healing rituals soon followed. In 1874, former
practitioners of Shugendō were prohibited from renting accommodations in
towns and calling them temples. They also could not use the title "Shugenja"
or don Shugendō robes.²⁷

Meiji officials justified the bans by claiming that *yamabushi*-type figures
spread "superstitions" (*meishin*), a newly coined term that literally meant
"belief gone astray."²⁸ The elimination of such wayward beliefs, officials and
others argued, was essential to demonstrating to Western powers that Japan
was worthy of joining the ranks of "civilized" nations. Superstitions supposedly deluded the populace and instigated social unrest, undermining efforts
to achieve "civilization and enlightenment." In newspaper reports of the
1870s and 1880s, rituals related to such supposedly wayward beliefs were
depicted as violent and harmful. In an 1877 article entitled "A Superstition
for Eliminating Fox-Spirit Attachment" in the *Yūbin hōchi* newspaper, one
reform-minded journalist recounted the story of a woman in Saitama prefecture whose neighbors tried to rid a fox spirit from her body.²⁹ When the
woman became delirious on the day of her husband's funeral, her neighbors
concluded that such delirium could only have resulted from fox- or racoon-
dog (*tanuki*)-spirit attachment. They called a Buddhist priest to perform
the fire ritual (*goma*) practiced in Shingon traditions, but when the measure
proved ineffective, they began to beat her, a common tactic for driving out
malign spirits. The newspaper reported that the widow tried to escape, all
the while babbling about a craving for fried tofu. The reporter criticized the
violent and abusive measures used to treat the woman's affliction, denouncing
the esoteric Buddhist rituals and beatings in a language resonant with that of
the anti-Buddhist edicts.

Religious specialists who performed ritual prayers (*kaji kitō*), too, were
maligned in newspaper reports that emphasized the "immoral" behavior of
religious healers. In one account in 1875, a journalist exhorted readers to refrain from hiring religious specialists who performed ritual prayers by relating
the story of Ikeda Tokujirō, a carpenter living in the neighborhood of Kanda
in Tokyo.³⁰ Ikeda's wife had "a beautiful face, but after giving birth, perhaps
due to *chi no michi* ('the path of blood') would say strange things and act as
if she were crazed from time to time."³¹ Believing that she was afflicted by a
fox spirit, her husband requested the services of a *hōin* named Asai, a member

of a Shinto sect called Ontake-kō. Asai agreed to perform ritual prayers, but prohibited anyone from entering the room where he was praying with Ikeda's wife, lest the entrants, too, became affected by the fox spirit. Asai's chants rang throughout the night. The next day all was quiet until Ikeda heard his wife suddenly cry out, "Don't do that!" Her husband quickly pulled open the screen door and found that Asai had climbed on top of his wife in a "lewd" manner. Her condition, the reporter lamented, deteriorated further thereafter.[32]

Newspaper accounts of persecution perpetuated the recurrent stereotype of religious and spiritual healers, whether clerics or practitioners, as swindlers who preyed on the populace through fees for ritual prayer and other services. But most clerics were not amassing wealth through the fees derived from these services in the mid- to late nineteenth century.[33] Likely many sought economic and social stability in the face of government proscriptions of long-standing religious institutions and practices. Many practitioners, especially *yamabushi*, also faced growing competition from newly emerging religious associations (later known as the New Religions) such as Kurozumikyō, Tenrikyō, and Konkōkyō for followers and their material resources. *Yamabushi* had long played key roles in family and communal religious life, even holding "parish" territories and managing Buddhist temples and Shinto shrines alongside their Shugendō temples. When their parishioners began to turn to the New Religions for various rites of health and healing, they lost crucial revenue.[34]

The Meiji government's efforts to legitimize its political rule by banning such religious practitioners as *yamabushi* and their rituals overlapped with another state-led project: the establishment of a centralized medical and public health system. One of the new regime's most pressing concerns from the 1870s onward was controlling the spread of such infectious diseases as cholera and syphilis, whose incidences surged with the opening of Japan's ports to trade with Europe and the United States.[35] The government elevated Western-derived medicine above what was starting to be called traditional Sino-Japanese or folk medicine by recruiting physicians trained in Dutch medicine in the late Edo period to establish national and prefectural medical schools. Beginning in the 1870s, government ministries assumed responsibility for administering all medical matters in the country, promulgating the Regulations on Medical Practice (*Isei*) in 1874 that established standards for medical education and a licensing system for physicians, pharmacists, and midwives. In the following years, various iterations of Bureaus of Hygiene (*eisei kyoku*) within the Home Ministry took charge of administering policies related to the regulation of physicians, the improvement of hygienic practices, the supervision of medical schools and hospitals, and the prevention and control of epidemics.[36] Academic psychiatry was established in medical schools as a result of such government funding and control of medical matters, as well as an increasing influence of German medicine in Japan.

Early Japanese psychiatrists contributed to Meiji government efforts to implement a new medical system and culture by redefining fox-spirit-related ailments as symptoms of "sickness of spirit" (*seishinbyō*), the literal Japanese translation of the German word *Geisteskrankheit*. Both terms are commonly translated into English as "mental disease" or "mental illness."[37] Psychiatrists reinterpreted fox attachment as mental illness as a means to establishing their new profession's authority. The redefinition project evolved from the late 1870s to the early 1900s, building on exchanges between local Japanese physicians and German doctors and then encompassing a wide range of research, from asylum-based empirical studies to ethnographic surveys.[38] It became the first major study by the first generation of Japanese psychiatrists in which they grappled with how to adapt allegedly universal categories of European psychiatry to explain such local phenomena as fox attachment.

As in other areas of medical knowledge, German physicians were highly influential in the field of Japanese psychiatry. Erwin Baelz, one of many German physicians hired by the Meiji state to teach and help build medical programs, became an authoritative source on the topic of fox attachment in the 1880s. Baelz came to Japan on a self-proclaimed civilizing mission. As he wrote in his diary in 1876 a few months before departing for Japan, "I am to play a part in the diffusion of western civilization among a gifted population eager for knowledge."[39] Once in the country, Baelz assumed the role of expert on matters related to animal-spirit possession in other areas of the world he considered peripheral, like India, Persia, China, and Palestine, where people suffered from a "confusion of voices" similar to cases of fox attachment in Japan. In 1885, Baelz published an article in several Japanese medical journals in which he explained that fox attachment was "a symptom of a mental defect" (*seishin shōgai shō*), which derived from a malfunction in which the two halves of the brain became independent from one another while continuing to perform their respective functions.[40] In a healthy person, only one half of the brain was actively engaged—in right-handed persons the left half of the brain, and in left-handed persons the right—while the other half contributed only in a general manner to the function of thought. "Nervous excitement" aroused the other half, Baelz explained, so that the two parts of the brain were set against one another. The fox therefore occupied the half of the brain that was not typically fully engaged and began to take on a life of its own.

The afflicted person, Baelz described, "hears and understands everything that the fox inside says or thinks; and the two often engage in a loud and violent dispute, the fox speaking in a voice altogether different from that which is natural to the individual."[41]

Around the time of Baelz's article, Japanese psychiatrists donned the cloak of ethnographers and traveled to rural areas of the country known for their shape-shifting foxes, racoon-dogs (*tanuki*), and dog-spirits (*inugami*). There they conducted surveys and administered medical examinations in order to collect data that would help build empirical foundations for further research on fox attachment. Kure Shūzō, who would be appointed chair of the Department of Psychiatry at Tokyo Imperial University in 1901 and become the most prominent psychiatrist of the pre-World War II generation, was especially keen on promoting the fusion of anthropological research and clinical observation. In the 1890s, Kure not only dispatched medical students to rural parts of the country to examine people afflicted by fox attachment, but also posted advertisements in medical journals asking for local doctors to send similar surveys to his department. Two such surveys were conducted in southwestern Japan: Shimamura Shun'ichi's 1891 survey of fox attachment in Shimane prefecture and Araki Sōtarō's 1900 survey of dog-spirit attachment in Tokushima prefecture.[42] Both men were medical students at the time who saw themselves as flag bearers of civilization and enlightenment. As Shimamura announced during a lecture at the Shimane Hygiene Association in 1891, "my humble wish is to do nothing else besides awaken the people from their delusions by assessing fox-spirit attachment from the perspective of psychiatry."[43]

Surveys of animal-spirit attachment by medical doctors would not have been possible without official state support. Local officials and physicians cooperated with Shimamura when he visited eastern Shimane in 1891. Upon arriving in the prefectural seat of Matsue, Shimamura called on Dr. Yamazaki Miki, the director of Matsue Hospital. Dr Yamazaki introduced him to Shinozaki Gorō, the prefectural governor, who promised the full support of his office. The prefectural office then sent an administrative order to every district office and district-level medical association, instructing local officials to report all persons believed to be suffering from fox attachment. Dr. Yamazaki and a member of the hygiene bureau of the prefectural office also personally accompanied Shimamura on his journey through the prefecture, helping him interview and conduct medical examinations of a total of thirty-four people. In the case of Araki Sōtarō in Tokushima prefecture, the details of the local support he received are not available, but Araki mentions in his final report that he conducted his investigation under "official government orders." Araki concentrated on areas famous for dog-spirit and racoon-dog attachment, such as the village of Ikeda in the district of Miyoshi, which, according to Araki, was especially well known as a "gathering place for dog-spirits."[44] When a person succumbed to any kind of sickness in this village of 4,848 people, whether a cold or an unknown ailment, residents reportedly attributed the illness to dog-spirits. In such areas that were steeped in the spirits of various animals, Araki examined twenty-one individuals over the course of three weeks.

The psychiatrist-ethnographers who descended upon rural villages wracked by spirit attachment diagnosed the afflicted along gendered lines. Interpreting fox attachment as a symptom of a specific disease, they determined that the afflicted men suffered from an array of ailments, including paranoia, mania, alcoholism, cholera, and typhus. Most of the women, on the other hand, were diagnosed with hysteria, a category beginning to appear in Japanese medical and popular discourses around this time. Although some Japanese medical studies attributed hysteria to both men and women, the psychiatric surveys of spirit attachment strongly associated the ailment with women.[45] Among the women examined by Shimamura and Araki, for instance, fifteen out of twenty-one and thirteen out of eighteen, respectively, were seen as having developed hysteria, while none of the men were diagnosed with it. Few medical specialists in Japan and elsewhere agreed on the origins, causes, and content of the disorder. In Europe, as historian Mark Micale has written, "nineteenth-century doctors hypothesized about whether hysteria derived from an anatomic lesion, a molecular change, a nutritional deficiency, or an electrophysiological irregularity in the brain." [46] But since their findings remained inconclusive, doctors were forced to define hysteria solely in terms of its symptoms, which they believed could be grouped into "symptom clusters" and then into discrete disease categories.

The psychiatric surveys suggested that fox attachment in women was a symptom of hysteria. Although the symptoms associated with hysteria changed over the years, in the 1870s and 1880s the diagnosis centered on the hysterical attack and the motor and sensory "stigmata," or signs of disease— paralyses, contractures, anesthesias, hyperesthesias, and dysfunctions of vision and hearing. According to influential nineteenth-century German psychiatrist Richard von Krafft-Ebing, whose work would profoundly influence that of the first generation of Japanese psychiatrists, people diagnosed with hysteria therefore experienced "extreme impressionability, extraordinarily intense reaction of the mind, and the rapid alternation of forms of excitement." In other words, patients of hysteria exhibited signs of "emotional anomalies," becoming extremely sensitive to internal and external psychic stimuli. Not only were patients unable to distinguish between imagination and reality, but they also supposedly experienced "illusions of cutaneous sensibility," falsely interpreting sensations on the skin.[47] Hysteria could therefore cause mistaken sensory experiences such as that of a fox spirit entering the body through one's fingernails.

The psychiatrists underscored women's experiences in their childhood and with their sexuality to arrive at the diagnosis of hysteria. After interviewing a sixteen-year-old unmarried woman, for instance, Shimamura concluded, "It is clear that she exhibits signs of hysteria, especially since when she was a child she suffered from 'nervousness' (*shinkeisei*) and in her adolescence she showed no signs of sexual desire (*tenki*)."[48] Shimamura considered the repeated spasms of pain in her abdomen to be symptoms of hysteria as well. The fever he attributed to rheumatism. The reason the young woman came to believe in fox attachment, according to Shimamura, was because she had heard as a child the "delusionary belief" (*mōshin*) that foxes could invade human bodies. In another instance, Shimamura diagnosed a woman who was struck with fox attachment at ages sixteen and nineteen as exhibiting "spasmodic hysterical psychosis" (*hossasei hisuterii-kyō*), explaining that she showed signs of having a "nervous disposition" (*shinkeishitsu*) as a child. Each time the woman was struck with spasms, she entered a state of agitation, which soon turned into a case of fox attachment.[49]

It is likely that Shimamura and Araki's surveys influenced later psychiatric interpretations of fox attachment in women. In 1902, psychiatrist Kadowaki Sakae diagnosed one third of the fifty-three women in his study of fox-spirit attachment cases at Sugamo Hospital with hysteria.[50] In 1905, Japanese psychiatrist Kure Shūzō affirmed the connection between hysteria and fox spirits in an article in a women's magazine: "It is very common that the nervous illness called *shaku* (癪) in the olden days, which is now known as 'hysteria,' is seen as fox attachment." According to Kure, people often confused hysteria for fox attachment because "if you become afflicted by [hysteria], your disposition (*seishitsu*) changes dramatically from its normal state." Kure further described how one could become extremely sensitive when suffering from hysteria, reacting severely to even the smallest thing, or become overjoyed and then just as easily angry, so that one day a person could be enjoying life and the very next she might be "swarmed by sadness." Kure claimed that when the emotions reached such extreme states, the body was affected by convulsions (*keiren*), known at the time as hysterical fits, hallucinations, and delusions.[51]

Psychiatrists redefined fox attachment as a symptom of gendered and sexualized illnesses like hysteria, offering a vision of minds and bodies that was radically different from that of the afflicted and their families. Symptoms of mental illness, they argued, derived from within the sufferer's mind and body, triggered by factors deemed internal to the individual such as family medical history, physiological abnormalities, sex, and personality. An individual's mind and body were no longer understood to be porous, but seemed instead to be self-contained and impenetrable to supernatural and social forces. Japanese psychiatrists would come to argue that the object of medical treatment was not a disease, but a person's "individuality," or the unique and personal set of circumstances and conditions of both mind and body that have created in a person some kind of disturbance or instability. As Kure Shūzō wrote in the introduction of the first major Japanese textbook of psychiatry:

> With regard to the treatment of mental illness (*seishinbyō*), one must realize that [it] is by no means to be treated as a single disease entity, but rather as a single individual who has an illness. It is most likely that the mental illness differs depending on the manifold illnesses of the organs, and is therefore [about] individuality. The essentials of treatment lie in the individual's medical history, the nature of the illness for the individual (*byōsei*), and the cause of illness.[52]

Historian Hyōdō Akiko has interpreted the newfound focus on the individual in psychiatry as part of a broader move toward a disciplinary regime of modernity that sought to pathologize the individual and his or her existence in an oppressive and reductive way.[53] She and others have suggested that psychiatrists discussed fox attachment as an issue of individual pathology at the expense of the social and communal contexts in which the cases occurred.

Indeed, those afflicted by fox spirits and their families understood experiences of attachment as embedded in social relations within and among families in villages. Psychiatrists may have dismissed such understandings, but their ethnographic surveys are brimming with anecdotes and other details that render visible the complexities of fox attachment against the background of ordinary village life. The details recorded in the surveys about petty disputes and grudges between neighbors, as well as the language used to describe the sufferings of spirit attachment, gesture toward a form of life that refused to be tamed by the universalist language of psychiatry.

Sticking to Families in Southwestern Japan

Although psychiatrists redefined fox attachment in the allegedly universal language of psychiatry, their ethnographic surveys and other materials confirm the localized and heterogeneous nature of the phenomenon. Consider the highly diversified lexicon used to describe foxes and their spirits. The standard word for fox was *kitsune*, but in southern Kyūshū it was known as *yako*, field fox, and in the Kantō region it was called *osaki*. In present-day Shizuoka, Nagano, and Yamanashi prefectures it was given the name of *kuda*, or "pipe [fox]." Under the name of *izuna*, it covered much of the Tōhoku district, and as *gedō*, meaning a Buddhist heresy, it appeared in the old province of Bingo in Hiroshima prefecture.[54] Foxes that roamed the ancient lands of Izumo in present-day Shimane prefecture were known in local lore as *ninko* or *hito-gitsune*, which literally meant "human-fox," and dogs, or dog-like foxes, found in Awa, the former name for an area of Tokushima prefecture, were called "*inugami*," or "dog-spirits."

Foxes across the country behaved—or were made to behave—in different ways, too. The psychiatric surveys confirmed that southwestern Japan's rural villages were known for something called "fox holding" or "fox ownership" (*kitsune mochi*), in which certain families were said to use foxes to inflict harm on neighbors. Villagers told psychiatrists that this practice of using foxes had a long history. In the provinces of Izumo and Awa, fox ownership allegedly originated in social tensions created by upheavals in village life in the eighteenth century. According to an account written in 1809 by a village headman named Yamane Yoemon, a wealthy farmer from the eastern Onshu district a century prior began to incur the resentment of his tenant farmers for levying heavy tributary taxes. One day, when a member of the wealthy farmer's family fell sick, one of the tenant farmers spread the rumor that a fox spirit had attached itself to the patient. The patient then started to act as if he were a fox, asking for tofu and red-bean rice.[55] The rumor soon spread that certain families owed their wealth and good fortune to the powerful foxes they owned. Foxes, after all, were known to be wily figures of deception. In this way, the fox acquired new symbolic meaning and uses as an instrument of village-level ostracism against those accused of fox ownership.

Accusations of fox ownership in the southwest regions of Japan from the eighteenth century on were connected to the economic and social transformations of the late Edo period.[56] New networks of commerce, trade, and culture had started to crisscross the country, integrating urban and rural economies in ways that fueled the growth of a new class of peasant landlords. As traders, moneylenders, and landowners, enterprising landlords accumulated wealth by taking advantage of new markets and amassing large plots of land to be distributed among small holders and tenant farmers, dramatically increasing the disparity in wealth between well-to-do and poor villagers. Resentment mounted among the vastly greater population of small holders, landless tenants, and laborers who lived in poverty and were at the mercy of their landlords, as well as famines and natural disasters.[57]

Families accused of owning foxes in the Edo period had usually been members of this growing class of peasant landlords. In a study of his own family's subjection to accusations of fox ownership since the early 1700s, Hayami Yasutaka explains that the Hayami family had been prominent titled peasants of Kanbara village, whose elevated social status had derived from family pedigree and support from feudal authorities in the sixteenth century. But when the family fell on hard times toward the end of the seventeenth century, another household from outside the village, moneylenders who had risen from obscurity, assumed the Hayami family name by legal adoption. The new family attempted to revive the older family's status in the village leadership, but they were opposed by the other "founding" peasant families (*kusawake hyakushō*) of the village, resulting in a conflict that stigmatized the Hayami family as fox owners and expelled them forever from village leadership positions.[58] Accusations of fox ownership therefore served as powerful weapons wielded by older, often impoverished "founding" families to protect their status and political power in the face of the incursions of new, wealthy families moving into villages and moving up the social ladder.[59] Families accused of fox ownership were stigmatized to the point of being disqualified for leadership in the village, and they were shunned by villagers who did not want to risk being identified as fox owners themselves.

By the time psychiatrists conducted their surveys of villages in Shimane prefecture and its surrounding areas in the 1890s and 1900s, some things had changed in the wake of Meiji government–led reforms. In 1887, a few former domains—the basic unit of provincial government in the Edo period—were consolidated and reorganized into the administrative unit of Shimane prefecture, with Matsue designated the capital city. New land tax reforms replaced the seigniorial control of arable land with private property rights, creating greater economic differentiation among farmers. In the 1880s, a massive reorganization of rural administration combined 79,000 villages across the country into some 14,000 larger villages in hopes of creating more fiscally sound units.

The redrawing of the administrative and political map of the region had limited impact on the everyday lives of residents, however. To the dismay of bureaucrats in the Home Ministry, old forms of organizations continued to prevail. The old villages, as historian Ann Waswo writes, "relegated to the status of hamlets and given no formal role in local government, [continued] to function as the primary sphere of the farmers' lives and the focus of their loyalties."[60] Many villagers regarded the new village to which they nominally belonged as an artificial institution and continued to turn to the hamlet for community. As the basic territorial units of society, hamlets consisted of interdependent households that were compelled to cooperate in order to survive. Farming continued to be a vulnerable occupation, and communal solidarity ensured survival. Specifically, farming families were compelled to maintain formal membership in hamlets, which continued to own two essentials of agricultural production: water for irrigation and forests for fuel, fodder, and green manure. Rights of access, and attendant obligations to share in its upkeep, could only be attained through formal membership in the hamlet. Throughout the newly created prefectures of Shimane and later Tottori, residents continued to live in small agricultural and fishing villages, many of them turning to sericulture and silk reeling in the early Meiji period as farming became increasingly costly and difficult.[61] Cooperation and communal solidarity among villagers ensured survival, making the inevitable competition and disruption all the more undesirable and important to quell.

The psychiatric surveys reveal the extent to which ideas and practices related to fox attachment were deeply embedded in patterns of village life. Given the etiquette and institutions of status inequality and hierarchy, open expression of grievances among villagers was virtually impossible, providing an opening for the spirits of foxes. When prompted by a religious healer or observer, the fox spirit that had adhered itself to a person might speak about the reasons for attachment, many of which concerned topics that most villagers would have found difficult to broach openly. Foxes, for instance, spoke often about problems caused by money, especially the borrowing and lending of money between neighbors.[62] One woman living in Shimane prefecture in May 1891 started to beg for red-bean rice cakes and red-bean rice while she lay suffering from fever, abdominal pain, headaches, and lockjaw.[63] Convinced that a fox spirit had attached itself to the woman, her parents pressed the fox to reveal the reason it had overtaken their daughter's body. After some cajoling, the fox replied: "I am a human-fox, and I have come from X's [name censored] house." When pushed further, the fox explained that it had come "due to a money issue." The father then suddenly remembered a debt of 50 *sen* that he had not paid back to a neighbor, someone known for his use of foxes.

Like money, fox spirits mediated social interactions between families in rural villages, bringing them into contact with one another even after death. In the village of Ikeda in Tokushima prefecture, a sixty-year-old widow was said to be afflicted with dog-spirits from two different dog-spirit-owning families.[64] The first family had borrowed money from the woman's husband when he was alive, but when she later demanded repayment of the loan, the family had threatened to unleash their dog-spirit on her. The second family had once sold firewood to another family, a deal for which the woman's husband had been the mediator. As the mediator, her late husband had agreed to pay for the firewood, but he neither had the full amount of 6 yen nor could pay interest. When he begged the family selling the firewood to refrain from charging interest, they refused and even threatened to sue if he did not eventually pay the full amount plus interest. Since the husband had paid only 2 yen of the debt before passing away, the woman afflicted with the dog-spirit believed that the family had used one of their dog-spirits to torment her. The woman believed her husband's past misdeeds were coming to haunt her in the form of animal spirits. In the afflicted woman's account of the second family, the dog-spirit speaking through her painted a distinctly sympathetic picture of the late husband, who had acted in a generous spirit to help his neighbor. The objects of resentment were the two dog-spirit-owning families, one of whom refused to repay a debt and the other who refused to forgive a 4-yen debt, both arguably breaches of neighborly duty and mutual obligation. Villagers like this afflicted woman invoked fox ownership and attachment to accuse others of unacceptable behavior.

Fox ownership persisted along familial lines in a way that conflicted with evolving Meiji ideologies and laws concerning family and kinship. Beginning in the 1870s, Meiji ideologues, government bureaucrats, legal scholars, and others promoted a structure of family organization and ideology known as the "*ie* system," which legalized and reinforced patrilineal primogeniture as the norm. But fox spirits were not easily assimilated into such a system. In the regions of Shimane and Tokushima prefectures, "fox ownership" and "dog-spirit ownership" were hereditary stigmas, passed down within a lineage and spread through marriage. Unlike the norm of patrilineal primogeniture, fox spirits traveled along matrilineal lines. A woman from a fox-owning family would allegedly bring foxes along with her. The stigma affected not only the individual household into which a woman married, but also the extended family of which it was a part, so that any man who married a woman from a fox-owning family was usually disinherited from his extended family. Indeed, in these areas of southwestern Japan, one of the first questions asked during the process of arranging a marriage was whether either family was a "fox owner."[65] Fox-owning families were known by a range of derogatory names, including *kuro* (black) and *warui hō* (wrong side), though they would not have been explicitly and publicly called such names. Men and women from such lineages were rarely accepted for marriage by non-fox-owning families, who designated themselves as *shiro* (white) or *yoi hō* (good side).[66]

The designations of "good side" and "wrong side" were not permanent. Bouts of madness could incite a family to accuse a "good side" neighboring family of owning foxes, as observed by the psychiatrists. When a seventeen-year-old man began to babble what seemed like nonsense, his father was convinced that their neighbor had unleashed foxes on him. Shimamura reported that the afflicted man was said to have declared: "I am a fox from the time of the Siege of Osaka. My name is Owasa. I am 360 years old. My parents are 500 years old."[67] The father then initiated a village-wide debate about the status of the neighboring family, gathering supporters to try to banish the allegedly fox-owning neighbor. In the end, the neighbors were allowed to remain after signing a "bond" document in which they agreed "not to unleash our foxes." It is possible that some prior friction between the two families incited one to accuse its neighbor of fox ownership. Whether a family could successfully "attach" the stigma of fox ownership to another family could depend on the assessment of the entire village. Accusations of fox ownership, which constituted a form of social discrimination, "stuck" only with communal agreement.

Foxes and dog-spirits also expressed the resentment and jealousy stirred up among families seeking marriage partners for their children, a social practice through which families and lineages became "attached" to one another.[68] A forty-eight-year-old woman named Ume in Tokushima prefecture, afflicted by a dog-spirit, spoke of a "black-haired woman from a dog-spirit-owning household." A public official named Sugiyama had apparently once considered the "black-haired woman" as a potential spouse, but then had started to court one of Ume's daughters. The "black-haired woman" had then used a dog-spirit to possess Ume, though she would have preferred to attack Sugiyama directly. The dog-spirit announced that it had indeed tried to bite and kill Sugiyama, but to no avail. In another village in Tokushima, a young woman noticed a pup (*inuko*) escape from the folds of her clothes and immediately thereafter began to experience bouts of spirit possession for over a year. During the third of five ritual prayers performed to exorcise the spirit, the dog-spirit revealed that it had come from a neighboring house known to be of "dog-spirit lineage" (*inugami suji*). The mother of the dog-spirit-owning family was said to be envious of the afflicted woman, whose beauty and health had attracted many suitors. The mother's own eighteen-year-old daughter, on the other hand, was "ugly and of stunted growth." The dog-spirit in a voice of its own said as much: "I've come from the neighboring house and I will stay here until their daughter is married." During the fifth prayer, the dog-spirit spoke once again: "I was told that I cannot return until the daughter is married."[69] In both accounts dog-spirit-owning and fox-owning matriarchs are represented as jealous, not because they were being discriminated against as fox-owning families, but because their own daughters were deemed less attractive as potential wives. Fox spirits evocatively mediated the matriarchs' struggles to create new kin on behalf of their daughters.

Jealousy regarding other people's wealth, even those within the same extended family, could elicit talk of fox ownership, too. Whereas stories from the Edo period emphasize fox-owning families being targeted for their newly accumulated wealth, the late nineteenth-century cases observed by Shimamura and other psychiatrists suggest that fox-owning families themselves could resent the industriousness of others. In one instance, when the family of an afflicted person asked the fox where it had come from, it replied: "I have come from the neighboring Yamamoto household. My house consists of five family members. Your family has only two or three people. Yet even when you are sick, you work in the fields. You strive to accumulate money and become rich. You are truly greedy. I see this from the side and there is no end to my feelings of jealousy. So I have come to attach myself to you." Or, jealousy could arise within families. One "patient" and her husband, as described by Shimamura, had been adopted into their impoverished family. The couple worked hard and succeeded in accumulating a few assets, but this made a relative envious. The unspecified relative then began to spread rumors about the couple being assisted by foxes as a way to explain their unexpected earnings.[70] Associating a part of the extended family with fox spirits thus created familial and social rifts.

When psychiatrists entered the world of "attachment" in rural southwestern Japan where fox spirits mediated such social practices as moneylending and marriage, their alternative diagnoses "stuck" only to varying degrees. Prefectural government officials, local doctors, and members of local medical associations welcomed the intervention of psychiatrists like Shimamura and Araki who conducted on-site medical examinations to confirm the theory that medical literature in circulation had already advanced: fox attachment was a symptom of various mental disturbances. This alternative explanation appealed to local officials and doctors for at least two reasons. For one, it incorporated their own prefectures into the greater nationwide project of "civilization and enlightenment," increasing the status of prefectures considered economic backwaters in peripheral areas of the country. It also helped to discredit the discrimination toward so-called fox-owning households, a social problem that had plagued the southwestern region since the eighteenth century. As the Shimane prefectural governor Shinozaki Gorō explained to Shimamura, the phenomenon of "human-foxes" did not simply affect an individual, but spread harm in society by establishing "strange customs" (*ki naru fūzoku*). Gorō claimed that even the slightest hint of fox ownership could ostracize a household indefinitely. When families entertained requests for marriage, for instance, the first item that they investigated was whether the household owned foxes. Gorō noted further that villagers who were identified as owning foxes were often forced to leave on pilgrimages or sometimes even committed suicide. For government officials like Goro, if psychiatrists could dispel the belief in fox spirits and fox ownership, they would help ameliorate a long-standing social problem. Local leaders were interested in the psychiatric intervention primarily because of its utility in serving local needs.

Among families most intimately affected by fox attachment, the psychiatric intervention "stuck" in curious ways. Some of the individuals and families examined by Shimamura and Araki seem to have found the new psychiatric explanation appealing for practical reasons of their own, rather than because they were convinced of the accuracy of the new diagnoses. Shimamura included in his report the reaction of a woman from the village of Shōbara who "left the [examination] room feeling quite joyous after understanding that I had diagnosed her with a mental illness, since she would no longer have to exhaust her assets in trying to get rid of the human-fox."[71] In other words, the woman's family would no longer feel compelled to pay for expensive religious healing rituals in order to exorcise the fox spirit. It is hard to determine how many others responded with relief to the diagnosis of mental illness, or even whether Shimamura had assessed her emotions accurately, but it is certainly possible that the woman embraced the doctor's diagnosis because it extended the practical benefit of eliminating a burdensome expense. The psychiatrist's explanation helped the woman with a practical issue, but it did not remove her from the world of "attachment." In fact, it further embedded her in that world with the new vocabulary of mental illness in hand. She had found a way to weave the psychiatric diagnosis into the language and logic of the world of fox attachment.

Shimamura and Araki's visits seem to have troubled local residents in Shimane and Tokushima prefectures for reasons unrelated to the new psychiatric diagnoses. Most families and individuals afflicted by fox attachment were unwilling to cooperate with the medical examinations and interviews because they did not want to publicize the condition. As Shimamura wrote, "many people tend to avoid telling others that he or she has the disease of fox attachment, making it difficult to conduct interviews."[72] The husband of the woman from Atsuhara village at first refused to send his wife to the local inn where Shimamura was conducting the interviews because he feared that such exposure would spread rumors about his family possibly using human-foxes. Such rumors would negatively affect his business, he declared. The involved parties came to a compromise and held the interview in the town hall. Still, Shimamura recorded in his report that the medical interview caused a commotion resembling a "sideshow" (*misemono*) as villagers gathered inside and outside the town hall, and eventually the police were forced to subdue the crowd so that the interview could continue. Although it is unclear whether villagers were curious about the afflicted individual, the doctor visiting from Tokyo, or both, it is telling that families did not resist Shimamura or his diagnoses, but rather feared the possibility of rumors about fox attachment affecting their household's reputation and livelihood. As soon as villagers heard the psychiatric diagnoses, they wove them into their everyday concerns. Psychiatric interventions "stuck" among rural residents once they were absorbed and then recast to address immediate problems, both within and beyond the village setting.

Expanding the Parameters of the Language of "Attachment"

As families and communities across nineteenth-century Japan confronted disruptions and contagions related to the global forces of imperialism, they expanded the parameters of the language of "attachment" to include not only animals and their spirits, but also new diseases. Shape-shifting animals were famously blamed for the cholera epidemics that swept through the country in the nineteenth century. Cholera originated in Bengal in 1817 and entered Japan through port cities such as Tsushima and Nagasaki, which were tied into trade networks with Europe, China, and Southeast Asia. The first pandemic hit the Osaka area in 1822, but remained geographically limited to the southwest of the country. But the second pandemic in 1858, carried by the US Navy from the coastal cities of China to Nagasaki, killed more than 800 in Nagasaki and reached the city of Edo, where in just two months it caused more than 30,000 deaths in a population of about one million. Cholera returned to Japan for a third time in 1877, and for the next two decades was semi-endemic, with over 200,000 deaths in 1879 and a similar number in 1886.[73] Before the Meiji government took control of the fight against the disease in the 1870s, villagers and urban residents for the most part were left to devise their own ways of figuring out the cause of the epidemic and fighting the disease with magico-religious talismans and herbal remedies.[74]

Terrified by the outbreaks of cholera, whose etiology confounded Japanese as it did many others around the world at the time, residents of rural areas fashioned theories about malicious foxes and dog-spirits roaming the countryside. The deaths were so mysterious that people like thirty-nine-year-old sake vendor Yahe'e of Ōmiya village in Suruga domain (present-day Shizuoka prefecture) recorded in his diary that on the evening of August 6, 1858, a neighbor named Kanegura died of the disease in such a "strange" (*fushigi*) way that the villagers believed it was the "deed of a fox" (*kitsune no waza*). Another villager, a female servant who fell ill that day, feeling a lump in the side of her stomach, cried out that a "pipe-fox" had attached itself to her. The pipe-fox was believed to be a microscopic creature slender enough to fit inside a small pipe that entered a person through a single pore of the skin.[75] Others believed that the fox was in fact an odd creature known as the "thousand-year mole." When the news of a humiliating treaty forced onto Japan by the United States and four European powers reached the village in 1858, the strangeness of the fox or mole quickly became associated with the strangers who had landed on Japan's shores. The creature spreading cholera, some villagers claimed, was the "American fox" (*Amerika gitsune*). Once a Dutch physician identified the devastating disease as cholera, which Japanese pronounced as *ko-re-ra* or *ko-ro-ri*, literate rural residents went so far as to attach the following animal *kanji*, or Chinese characters, to the word: fox for *ko*, wolf for *ro*, and raccoon-dog (*tanuki*) for *ri*, or 狐狼狸. One spelling of the word for cholera thus literally meant "[the work of] foxes, wolves, and raccoon-dogs."[76]

Families also invoked the language of fox attachment when managing social and institutional changes of the early Meiji years. In the case of a young man named Yoshirō from a village in Kanagawa prefecture, for instance, his family's invocation of fox attachment contained a subtle critique of the newly established military conscription. As reported in the national *Yomiuri* newspaper in 1880, Yoshirō, a recent conscript, became so anxious about the possibility of being killed in battle that he began to act "a little crazed," eventually locking himself up in his room.[77] Yoshirō's breakdown occurred only a few

years after the promulgation of the Conscription Act of 1873, an unprecedented measure that made military service a national duty for all men between
the ages of seventeen and forty. The act evoked hostile responses all over the
country in the form of widespread draft evasion and even armed uprisings.
Yoshirō was thus not alone in his anxiety. But Yoshirō's older brother confi-
dently determined that Yoshirō was suffering from fox attachment. His sister,
Yahachi, then had what the reporter describes as an "absurd thought" but was
a well-known local cure for fox attachment: that the best way to force the
fox to leave was by pointing a gun toward it. She packed a bamboo pipe with
gunpowder and held it under Yoshirō's nose, calling "come out, come out" to
the fox. But no fox emerged, so she lit one end of the pipe with an incense
stick, causing the gunpowder to be blown out of the other end, and injuring
her left elbow.

In the midst of the commotion caused by the explosion, Yoshirō suddenly
began to talk, claiming to have been a fox for the past ten years. His family
then decided to send him to the local Shinto shrine to receive ritual prayers.
In the middle of the prayers, the village head (*kochō*) arrived on the scene to
admonish Yoshirō for trying to avoid his military duty. The village head, like
other town and village mayors, was required to serve on the local military
affairs board and was therefore responsible for seeing that the young men
under his jurisdiction registered as conscripts and cooperated with a process that imposed hardships and brought no visible benefits to the residents
of the town or village.[78] "It is too bad," concluded the reporter, "that un-
fortunately Yoshirō will probably be attacked and killed," implying that he
would lose his life as a soldier in battle. Although the article suggested that
Yoshirō was trying to evade conscription under the guise of being afflicted
by a fox, the reporter also expressed sympathy for Yoshirō's fate as a newly
conscripted soldier.

Popular representations of fox-spirit attachment, too, invoked families
in ways that prompted viewers to consider the nature and consequences
of various forms of "contact." In 1885, artist Ochiai Yoshi'iku, for instance,
created a woodblock print based on a previously published newspaper article (*shinbun nishikie*) about a merchant in Yokohama whose family became
convinced that his bouts of babbling were "the workings of a *tsukimono*," or
a spirit that had attached itself.[79] The print shows a gathering of seven men
turned toward a man with the face of a fox sitting on some bedding, with
a woman holding an infant nearby. The text surrounding the image, which
partially reproduced that of the original newspaper article, explained that
the fox-faced man was the merchant being treated for spirit-attachment. His

family had decided to summon the leader of a pilgrimage group associated with a holy mountain, who had arrived at the merchant's home with five or six fellow members of the pilgrimage group to conduct the usual rituals. The leader prayed, lit a fire, and rang bells, but the merchant seemed unaffected. So he began physically beating the afflicted man, a common method of driving out spirits, but the "sick person" (*byōnin*) could not tolerate the pain. "Thinking he could momentarily escape the pain [of the beating] by pretending that a spirit had attached itself to him (*tsukimono no maneshite*), [the merchant] cried 'I'm leaving now!'" At that point the pilgrimage group leader asked the spirit for proof of its departure. The patient, "pretending to be the spirit," said he would leave behind three strands of red hair. "Everyone in the room creeps closer to the patient's bedside, but when the patient does not produce the strands of hair, the [pilgrimage group] leader orders the men to tie up the patient for another beating." Dreading another beating, the merchant jumped up and shouted, "Calm down and listen! An illness called syphilis is attached (*tsukete iru*) to my body. Nothing other than [syphilis] is attached. You all are the ones who have been duped by a fox or racoon-dog, making me, on top of everything else, perform useless and idiotic stunts." He then threatened to report them all to the Kanagawa Prefectural Office, which frightened the leader and his men. With awkward expressions on their faces, they left.

It might be tempting to interpret Ochiai's print as aiming to disabuse viewers of the notion of fox-spirit attachment. After all, the merchant seems to enlighten the pilgrimage group leader and members that his symptoms derive not from an allegedly supernatural cause like fox-spirit attachment but from syphilis.[80] But even as the merchant reveals the "actual" cause of his condition, he deploys a playful and provocative language of "attachment" that complicates binaries of supernatural and natural, unreal and real. He describes syphilis as being "attached" to his body, in the same way that a fox spirit might be attached. Nor does he reject the possibility of shape-shifting animals adhering to humans, for he turns the table on the men by declaring that they are "the ones who are duped (*tsumamarete iru*) by a fox or racoon-dog." The repetition of verbs like "dupe" and "pretend," as in the man with a fox face "pretending" to speak like a fox spirit, suggests that no one can be sure who has the strongest claim on what is "actually" happening. The print plays with ideas of mimicry. When the fox-faced man imitates the voice and antics of a fox spirit, it generates ridicule and entertainment, but also uncertainty and discomfort. If a man infected with syphilis babbles nonsense to the point that those around him thinks that he is afflicted by a fox spirit, one might say

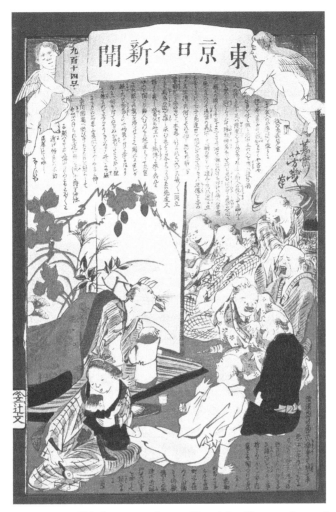

FIGURE I.I Yokohama merchant afflicted by "fox attachment." Ochiai Yoshi'iku, *Tokyo nichi nichi shinbun* 914 (January 23, 1885). Reproduced by permission from The Protected Art Archive / Alamy Stock Photo.

that the symptoms of syphilis can mimic those of fox attachment, making the two ailments indistinguishable from one another.

The syphilis in Ochiai's print conjures a form of contact that was known to harm families. Contemporary viewers would have immediately understood the significance of the presence of the woman with an infant in her arms. She is likely the wife of the merchant, who has been made susceptible, along with her child, to "the poison," as syphilis was commonly called. Viewers would have assumed that her husband had contracted syphilis after frequenting "the pleasure quarters." Although syphilis was a venereal disease that had existed in Japan since at least the sixteenth century, it spread rapidly with the increase in prostitution around ports like the one in Yokohama that opened to Euro-American powers in the mid-nineteenth century. Syphilis spread to such a degree that in 1871 the Council of State ordered the Home Ministry to require prefectural governments to establish examination centers for syphilis. The ensuing directive blamed the increase in prostitution for encouraging "men in their prime [to] fall into indolence and extravagance such that their businesses fail and their families are ruined. Moreover, many have contracted syphilis and become physically deformed, and then even spread the disease to their descendants."[81] Popular public health manuals and newspaper articles, too, repeated such warnings about the risk of intergenerational contagion. Indeed, the merchant's fox face evokes the possibility of deformation. If the syphilis that has "attached" itself to the merchant's body is manifesting itself by distorting his face into that of a fox, then the merchant's child, too, is at risk of such physical transformation. In a world of "attachment," syphilis appears as an ailment that adheres to families.

The state and psychiatric attack on ideas and practices related to fox spirits indirectly targeted long-established structures and cultures of care centered on the family. The Meiji state's ban on some forms of religious healing, especially those related to the exorcism of spirits, stemmed from its desire to assert political authority in the wake of the collapse of the Tokugawa regime and resulted in criticisms of the most common form of treatment for physical, mental, and spiritual afflictions available to families. Psychiatrists joined the campaign against fox spirits to support state efforts at overhauling long-standing cultures of healing and health, which then helped reinforce their own profession's claim that fox-spirit attachment was nothing other than a manifestation of gendered forms of "mental illness" or, to translate their term more literally, "sickness of spirit"—an ironic term given that the psychiatrists were trying to undermine notions of attaching spirits.

Yet the state and psychiatric projects of redefinition helped create an archive of materials that evocatively gestures toward the persistence and power of shape-shifting fox spirits in changing village and global circumstances of the late nineteenth century. As a mode of filiation that perpetuated lineages and shaped kinship ties, fox attachment continued to affect families in some villages, especially those in southwestern Japan. This mode of filiation was not seen by affected families simply as an "alternative" to the normative model of kinship based on ties of blood, biology, or law that hardened in the context of the creation of the Civil Code of 1898 and other ideologies of family from the 1890s onward. Matrilineal kinship as evoked by fox ownership practices, for instance, had long lived a layered existence with other forms and processes of filiation. *Tsuki* can thus offer a metaphor with which to conceptualize the nature of stasis and change across the Tokugawa and Meiji periods without resorting to binary models of the co-constitution of the old and the new. The metaphor of surface-level adherence and attachment calls attention to the piecemeal, temporary, and inconsistent ways in which ideas, people, and practices might "stick" to one another in one localized and ordinary moment, only to separate in another.

The persistence of fox spirits speaks to the continuing centrality of family, too. Although the early Meiji state and psychiatrists attempted to dismantle some structures and cultures of family-based care, they soon faced the material reality that an overhaul of the health, medical, and spiritual cultures in place would require tremendous resources that the state was not necessarily willing to provide. Indeed, in order to avoid paying for a social welfare system, the state would come to harness the power of family-based care and responsibility. It created new laws, ideologies, and structures of rule that further intensified family responsibility for those considered mentally and spiritually disturbed, a responsibility that the women in families would disproportionately bear.

2

Cages in Rural Homes

IN THE FALL of 1900, a wealthy farmer from Ōka village in Shizuoka prefecture, who had once occupied the eminent position of village headman,
began "inflicting problems" on his family and neighbors. He became "destructive" and "violent," according to a summary of statements given by his
wife to a visiting psychiatrist twelve years later. Although the specific ways in
which he may have been destructive and violent were not recorded, his behavior was disturbing and unpredictable enough for his family to resort to what
many rural residents had done since the preceding Edo period (1603–1868) to
restrain mentally disturbed members prone to violence: they received permission from local officials to confine the farmer in a narrow wooden enclosure
built inside the house. There the farmer would spend his days, his left leg in
chains and his sensations dulled to the point that he stopped speaking. A similar fate would befall the farmer's twenty-five-year-old son in the summer
of 1910, when he locked himself up in his room and fell into a deep depression. His condition rapidly deteriorated. According to his older brother, the
family decided to confine him, too, in a cage-like room after they found him
smearing his own excrement on his clothing and bedding. Like his father, he
was enchained inside the room so that he would not hurt himself. But unlike his father, he was not silent. He sang songs loudly, the sound of his voice
drifting through the wooden bars of his confinement room and reaching the
ears of those living with him in the house.[1]

The Ōka village family entered the historical record at a time when medical, legal, and governmental interest in regulating the long-standing practice of home confinement intensified. By the turn of the twentieth century,
the limits of state-led medical reforms had become clear. Meiji officials had
aspired to implement a far-reaching medical system of licensed Western-
trained physicians and hospitals that would become the dominant form of

Madness in the Family. H. Yumi Kim, Oxford University Press. © Oxford University Press 2022.
DOI: 10.1093/oso/9780197507353.003.0003

treatment for those who were physically and mentally ill, but the monetary cost of sweeping institutional change proved too onerous. To avoid the costs of a state-funded welfare system, Meiji politicians and lawmakers instead harnessed the power of such existing practices as home confinement to assert the family as the provider of care for members and relatives who were indigent, ill, or otherwise incapacitated. With the passage of the Civil Code of 1898 and the first national law concerning the confinement of the mentally ill in 1900, home confinement became subject to police and bureaucratic surveillance. Since at least the eighteenth century, families had been required to obtain permission from such local authorities as village- and neighborhood-based elders and leaders to use confinement rooms. From the 1870s onward, families reported instead to newly created local police and the prefectural governor, who in turn strove to ensure that families followed the terms of the new national laws regulating familial responsibility and home confinement. The new laws reflected conservative Meiji ideologies of the patriarchal family, increasing the legal and social powers of male household heads over women, children, and other dependents. Lawmakers, politicians, and bureaucrats saw an opportunity to reinforce this patriarchal vision in the regulation of home confinement.

Accounts of home confinement tend to focus on the ways in which the practice became an object of official surveillance, psychiatric intervention, and bureaucratic regulation at the turn of the twentieth century.[2] This is not surprising, given that the archive consists mostly of legal, medical, police, and bureaucratic records.[3] Under the new laws, families submitted written requests to the local police and prefectural governor that provided details such as the reasons for home confinement, the physical dimensions of the cage-like rooms, and the measures in place to ensure hygienic conditions. Once the room was built, national and prefectural laws required police to inspect it once or twice a month. Beginning in the 1900s, psychiatrists used the police records as a basis for finding families living with confinement in rural areas and conducted ethnographic surveys that yielded statistics, floor plans, photographs, interviews, and drawings of their conditions.[4]

Missing from analysis is a crucial factor that made home confinement possible in the first place: a domestic and moral economy of caregiving that heavily relied on women's physical and mental labor. In the case of the Ōka village farmer and his son, for instance, the extensive physical, mental, and emotional labor performed mostly by the women in the family ensured that the two men would survive confinement with as much dignity as the circumstances allowed. When the son soiled his clothing and bedding, it was

most certainly his mother or other female help who cleaned them. When father and son needed to eat, it was women in the family who prepared their
meals and even hand-fed them. This is not to say that their brother or other
male relatives were not involved at all in the labor of caregiving, but the
laboring hands of women are imprinted on the various documented cases
more so than those of men. Wives, mothers-in-law, husband's sisters, female
servants, and nursemaids contributed to the daily care of the confined, while
they also tended to the farm work, shop-keeping, cooking, cleaning, child
rearing, and other forms of reproductive and productive labor that sustained
the lives and livelihoods of their families. Yet their labor has remained too
ordinary and too self-evident to merit investigation as an enabling condition
of home confinement.

Centering women's everyday labor in an account of home confinement
illuminates the complexities and contradictions of family-based "care" for
those considered mad. Most families confined their mentally disturbed
member for fear of the trouble they caused (or might cause) other household
members, neighbors, and the wider village or neighborhood. Ideas about confinement as a mode of moral rehabilitation that originated in the preceding
Edo period lingered into the nineteenth and twentieth centuries. As a practice in which punishment, protection, and rehabilitation overlay one another,
home confinement rendered ambiguous the nature of the daily "care" that
women in families provided. Far from simply the provision of what was necessary for the health and maintenance of an afflicted person, "care" in the
context of home confinement was often hard to distinguish from abuse and
abandonment. When wives, sisters, elderly mothers, and daughters passed
food through the bars of a confinement room to the mentally afflicted relative, for instance, they nourished the bodies of the confined for the day but at
the same time increased the chances of death, since keeping people in confinement for long periods was often lethal.

Tending to the needs of the confined was often so arduous for women
caregivers that it attenuated kinship ties, even though the practice was
premised on the allegedly natural strength of family bonds. Indeed, the work
of women unsettled notions of the stable and natural ties of family touted by
state ideologues and new laws, showing instead the ways in which kinship was
contingent upon the provision of care in all its ambiguous and contradictory
forms. Through domestic acts of caregiving often rendered negligible or even
invisible by observers, women sutured the wounds inflicted by forms of madness. Such acts involved mediating institutional and intimate worlds, too. The
reality of caregiving at times rendered institutional directives meaningless.

Laws intended to put male household heads in charge became futile when it was usually men who were confined at home, compelling women in families to serve as legal guardians who tended to all interactions with the police, doctors, and other local authorities, as well as assume financial responsibility. Women's work sustained the very families on which the state relied as the alleged moral foundation of society. By making "the family" responsible for the care and custody of those considered mad, the state effectively shifted a disproportionate amount of the burden onto women.

Origins of a Domestic Culture of Confinement

Home confinement originated in the Edo period as a form of discipline and punishment directed at disobedient—but not necessarily mad—family members, which would eventually be adopted by early twentieth-century families confining those considered mad. One of the most common targets of confinement in the Edo period was the "profligate son" (*hōtō musuko*), whose father would throw him into a *zashikirō*, or "parlor prison," a formal sitting room turned into a prison-like cell, either by replacing the sliding doors with wooden bars or constructing a wooden cage inside the room.[5] Fathers hoped that restricting their sons' movements would compel them to reflect on past indiscretions and resolve to mend their ways. The low-ranking samurai Katsu Kokichi, forced to return home after having run away, found that "a cage (*ori*) the size of three tatami mats had been set up in the middle of the sitting room (*zashiki*)."[6] As Katsu relates in his autobiography of 1843, he lived inside the cage for three years, following his father's instruction to "think long and hard about [his] life."[7] Sons who served time in parlor prisons were usually from the samurai class or wealthy commoner families who could afford to hire carpenters to construct cages and delegate the task of feeding and caring for the son to a female servant in the household. Spaces of domestic confinement came to be associated with the pacification and moral reform of privileged but unruly young men.[8]

Literary and imaginative accounts of the eighteenth and nineteenth centuries, too, abounded with allusions to sons serving time in parlor prisons. Here confinement operated as a literary trope that expressed the relationship between space, body, and moral reform. As in the case of the samurai Katsu, it was assumed that behavior could be corrected by restricting a person's movement to a physically narrow space in which he was left with no choice but to reflect on his past actions. A well-known example can be found in "The Cauldron of Kibitsu" ("Kibitsu no kama"), a story from Ueda Akinari's *Tales*

of Moonlight and Rain (Ugetsu monogatari) (1776). Set in the sixteenth century, it tells the tale of a wronged wife who dies and haunts her husband and
his lover in the form of a vengeful possessing spirit. Early in the story, Shōtarō,
who is married to the faithful and steadfast Isora, is locked up in a *zashikirō* by
his father after he begins to spend days away from home with Sode, a woman
from the pleasure quarters. Shōtarō deceives Isora and runs away with Sode.
Isora, overwhelmed with distress and resentment, falls ills and dies, only
to track down and take revenge on her unfaithful husband and his lover.
Neither bodies nor emotions can withstand containment of any kind in this
story: Shōtarō breaks free of his cage, not to mention his familial obligations,
to abscond with his lover to another village, and Isora's resentment lives on
in the form of a malignant spirit even after her bodily death. Akinari's story
suggests that keeping the body in check—either in a cage or by death—does
little to restrain such strong emotions as desire and vengeance.

Fathers confined their sons, but mothers bore the guilt—or so the amateur poetry of the times suggests. Parlor prisons were a recurring theme
in a popular genre of poetry known as *senryū*, or short poems that gave
glimpses into everyday life and human nature with all their shortcomings and
idiosyncrasies. Often tinged with dark humor and cynicism, though not entirely devoid of light remarks and witty turns of phrase, *senryū* were written
mostly by amateur poets. In one of the most famous Edo-period collections,
The Willow Barrel (Haifū yanagidaru), a multivolume collection of poems
written by anonymous residents of the city of Edo between 1765 and 1838,
there are at least thirty-eight *senryū* that allude to parlor prisons.[9] Among
them, one recurring figure is the mother in despair at the sight of her confined
son. The confinement was seen as evidence of a mother's failure to raise her
son properly, so her agony was directed not only at her son, but also at her
own perceived inadequacy, as seen in the following three poems:

> *Parlor prison—*
> *There are mothers, too, in manacles*[10]

> *Parlor prison—*
> *A letter arrives*
> *And a mother's failure*[11]

> *Parlor prison—*
> *A mother's short-sleeved kimono*
> *Also a binding rope*[12]

The poems touch on the anguish of mothers who find themselves "in manacles," attesting to their shared experience of a son's confinement. It was not only the confined son who suffered, but his mother as well, for she was seen as bearing at least partial responsibility for her son's misdeeds. In the second poem, the letter was likely sent by a woman of the pleasure quarters.[13] Out of habit, the mother passed the letter to her son inside the parlor prison, evoking the act that led her son to squander his time in the pleasure quarters, which then landed him in the cage. A mother's sense of guilt might even impel her to turn her short-sleeved kimono into a rope used to bind criminals (*shibarinawa*) and kill herself, as in the third poem.

In popular imagination, the most common behavior punished by home confinement was wasting time and money in the pleasure quarters, common among samurai and wealthy commoners. A young man returns home in the morning from Yoshiwara, and is surprised to find a cage in the sitting room:

> *Returning home in the morning*
> *In the sitting room*
> *Is Denmachō*[14]

The sitting room has become the Denmachō Jailhouse, the main prison in the city of Edo established in the early 1610s.[15] Or, a parlor prison poem could suggest another kind of transformation:

> *A parlor prison*
> *In place of a bucket on the head*[16]

A bucket on the head refers to *okebuse*, a form of punishment directed at customers who did not pay for services in the pleasure quarters. The customer was forced to walk around the streets with a bucket on his head, a section of it carved out so that passersby could see his face. Both poems achieve rhetorical and emotional force through the ironic imposition of public forms of punishment—namely, bucket-covered heads and the city jailhouse—onto the intimate space of the family sitting room. Public and domestic spaces are unexpectedly conflated. Yet the blurred boundary between public and domestic spaces existed only in the world of metaphor. Public authorities and institutions such as constables or the jailhouse had nothing to do with the caging of wayward sons. Such was not the case for the confinement of family members who were considered mad.

The domestic confinement of a member deemed "mad" or "insane" required verification and permission from a range of authorities outside the family, regardless of where the afflicted person would be confined. Edo-period families usually chose one among three places to restrain a mad member prone to violence or other disruptive behavior: in a local prison (*jurō*), in a detention center (*tame*), or at home.[17] Placement in a local prison was bureaucratically the least complicated route. All that was required was the written agreement of the immediate family and the "five-household group" (*gonin gumi*), a communal association collectively responsible for paying taxes, preventing offenses against the law, providing one another with mutual assistance, and keeping a general watch over one another. One member's offense against public order, whether it involved charging more than the lawful price for a pack-horse or wearing inappropriately costly clothing, could result in the punishment of all members of the five-household group. Such collective liability meant that a family often placed those considered mad and prone to violence in local prisons as a preventative measure that would shield the group from vicarious punishment.

Similarly, the second method of confinement was *tame-azuke*, or the safe-keeping of an insane person at a detention center (*tame*). *Tame-azuke* was used primarily for those already confined in a local prison where conditions deteriorated to the point of causing unrest in the prison. He or she was then sent to a detention center used mostly to confine minor offenders and sick prisoners. In the city of Edo, the detention centers were located in Asakusa and Shinagawa, with a specially designated area (*ken*) within the center for the confinement of the mentally ill.[18] In cases of placement in local prisons or detention centers, the line between prevention and punishment, safekeeping and restraint blurred. Individuals were not placed in local prisons or detention centers as punishment, but the physical structure and original uses of the spaces as punitive sites made it difficult to disassociate confinement from punishment.

Of the three methods of managing those among the mentally disturbed who were prone to violence or other disruptive behavior, home confinement occurred the least frequently and required the most official oversight. As a section on enclosures for those considered mad in a handbook consulted by the rural magistrate of Nihonmatsu domain indicates, families were required to submit a request to confine at home only when "there is a mad person (*ranshinsha*) who cannot be left unattended in the village."[19] Among those who could not be "left unattended" and were therefore confined at home, most were individuals with senior status in the family, namely parents, grandparents, uncles, and heirs. In a society abiding by notions of familial hierarchy determined by age and gender, it was difficult to subject family elders to treatment that resembled disciplinary action in a public space such as the local prison or detention center. Persons of elevated status within families therefore tended to be confined at home.[20] A man whose name appears as "Seibei" in inspection documents, for instance, was an uncle in his adopted household in Asakusa in the city of Edo who was placed into confinement. In the documents his family declared that Seibei ought to be placed in prison, "but because he is an elder (*me ue no mono*) it is difficult to send him away [and] therefore [we request] permission to put him in a cage inside the residence. If this matter concerned a person of lesser standing (*me shita no mono*), one would have proceeded accordingly [i.e., sent him to a prison]."[21]

Home confinement entailed a complicated bureaucratic procedure that ensured that families, communal associations, and officials had all verified the condition of the afflicted person and approved confinement at home. The few extant records of Edo laws and provisions concerning those deemed mad indicate that at least five different groups of people were involved in the process of requesting and obtaining permission to confine at home: the family, relatives, the five-household group, village elders in the countryside or neighborhood chiefs in cities, and the rural district or city magistrate. At times a physician's diagnosis was also required. As guidelines written in 1814 for Edo city magistrates state, the first step in the permissions procedure was taken by members of the extended family when they collectively declared that a member was mad: "Parents and siblings, as well as relatives, should decide whether [this is a case of] madness, and obtain endorsement from a city or neighborhood official."[22] The official was usually the neighborhood chief in cities like Edo, who worked at the level closest to commoners. One of his duties was "to verify the accuracy and procedural correctness of petitions, complaints, and reports drafted by merchants and artisans for submission to the [city] magistrates, attested to by the chief's personal seal affixed to the back of the document."[23] The neighborhood chief or his representative would visit the petitioning family to conduct an inspection and then forward the request to his direct superior, one of the city elders. A city elder would then submit the proper documentation, usually including a sketch of the layout of the residence and projected location of the cage, to the city magistrates. The magistrate often sent out his own representative to inspect the residence and afflicted person as well, only then granting permission to confine. The sequence of persons consulted reflects the hierarchy, in reverse order, of the institutions that governed the lives of commoners in the Edo period. Representatives from each part of this clear structure of authority were expected to agree on and verify the madness (*ranshin*) of the individual in question.

Officials at all levels had a vested interest in requiring multiple points of verification of madness: they sought to prevent household strife that might produce grievances leading to the dissolution of a household. Dissolution meant one fewer taxable unit and one more source of social and economic instability. Since all shogunal domains taxed commoners to support samurai, domain officials took notice of commoner behavior when it affected the ability or willingness to remit taxes. With home confinement of the insane, domains were concerned about the possibility of household strife that might impede one specific and crucial event: succession of the household head.[24] If a current household head or his heir was deemed insane and confined to a room, the extended family, often in consultation with village heads, would designate another person as household head. No doubt tensions and conflicts ensued during the process of choosing a new household head while the former head sat caged inside his own house.

Families were invested in ensuring a smooth succession for the sake of domestic stability, but they were also aware of the need to convince authorities that the necessary precautions regarding potential succession and inheritance disputes had been taken. In a 1793 request for permission submitted to the city magistrate in Edo city to confine a pawnshop owner and household head in the neighborhood of Kanda, the families first addressed the issue of potential disputes. In the first of six documents submitted in July, the petitioner, who was the pawnshop owner's mother, affirmed that since becoming mentally disturbed her son had "shaved his head and changed his name to Tenjun," meaning that he had shed his former duties to become a monk with a Buddhist name. "In regards to the family estate," she continued, "we have the name of my grandson written as the successor," explaining that the pawnshop owner's fourteen-year-old son was to become the new owner and successor.[25]

But families were often compelled to confine by more immediate concerns than those related to succession. In the same 1793 petition concerning the Kanda pawnshop owner, his mother explained that her son's condition had made him "violent" and that he was disturbing the daily operations of the business. She reported that he was throwing household items and beating his wife and employees. Their decision to place him in confinement at home thus stemmed in part from the need to protect those around him from physical abuse. The potential negative impact on the five-household group and other neighbors factored into the family's decision, too. As in most Edo-period requests for home confinement, the official reason given in the petition was the phrase, "the source of fire is insecure." This standard phrase expressed the need to monitor a person so that he or she would not cause a fire or other accidents that might endanger the household and neighborhood. In densely populated towns and cities where the most common building material was wood and such features of houses as sliding doors were made of paper, fires spread quickly and could be devastating. Residents feared that those considered both mentally disturbed and uncontrollable might unintentionally cause fire, even when confined, which might result in penalties and punishment for the family and five-household group.[26] The terms of confinement as well as the extent of daily surveillance were thus relatively strict.

From its origins, home confinement was infused with complex and contradictory associations. Its connection to moral and physical rehabilitation, as when used with the disobedient sons of privileged Edo-period families, would continue to inform the practice into the twentieth century when families often assumed that violent behavior, even that of a member who had gone mad, could be "domesticated," or brought under control at home. At the same time, cages built inside the home resembled the spaces of local prisons and detention centers, suggesting that home confinement was a form of punishment for both potential and actual misdeeds and misbehaviors. Still, the desire to protect the mentally disturbed member and those around him or her continued to be a powerful source of motivation to confine. Whether to ensure the safety of family members, employees, neighbors, or the afflicted person, confinement was a practical, if extreme, measure taken by families. Official interest in regulating home confinement intensified in the mid-Meiji period as the new regime created laws and institutions concerning the welfare of those considered mad or otherwise incapacitated, ensuring that the central site of caregiving would remain the home, with all its attendant ambiguous and contradictory associations.

Layers of "Care" in Police Surveillance and the Law

In the early Meiji years, government officials, legal scholars, and psychiatrists' collective interest in managing the care and custody of mentally disturbed people produced competing and contradictory understandings of "care." Meiji officials sometimes cast their interest in controlling and monitoring the movements of those considered mad and socially disruptive in the language of care. When they assigned newly created prefectural police to replace the neighborhood heads and city magistrates to monitor those considered mad, the police conceived of themselves as "caretakers" of the new citizen-subjects of Japan. The Metropolitan Police Office of Tokyo, established in 1874 in the Home Ministry, played an unprecedented role as caretaker and guardian of the public peace, managing many aspects of daily life in the new capital city. Although technically responsible for security maintenance only in Tokyo, the Metropolitan Police Office quickly became the model for police systems in other prefectures. The nearly 6,000 newly recruited patrolmen were assigned a broad range of duties, from supervising commercial activities and conducting population counts to preserving public morals and compiling information on residents of each neighborhood. No other security institution in Japan had ever been so large or far-reaching. The police carried out paternalistic measures of preventive policing, recording and punishing ordinary people's customs and habits for the sake of stifling social unrest. As Kawaji Toshiyoshi famously wrote in *Keisatsu shugan* (1876), a widely read guide for policemen, "A nation is a family. The government is the parents. Its people are children. The police are their dry nurse."[27] In considering the police the "dry nurse" of the people, Kawaji feminized the police as caretakers of babies and children who served the supposed best interests of the latter.

When the Metropolitan Police office took over the administration of home confinement in the 1870s, their foremost concern was maintenance of the public peace during a time of political regime change. Such maintenance entailed removing persons deemed socially disruptive and unsightly from public view, especially during visits by foreign dignitaries or public parades conducted by the Meiji emperor. As early as 1874, the police issued an ordinance that ordered families to watch strictly over any members considered mad, and in May 1878 it announced the first major directive aimed at "caring for insane persons (*fūtennin,* 瘋癲人) and controlling wayward children":

> Those who have no choice but to confine at home (*shitaku*) in order to care for (*kango*) an insane person (*fūtennin*) or discipline a wayward child must first send to the ward chief a detailed description of the reason for confinement signed by two family members (and in the case of a mentally ill person a doctor's diagnosis form as well), in accordance with the procedure for placing in a cage [those who require reform] as outlined in the March 10, 1876 police ordinance, and then receive permission from the police office in the appropriate jurisdiction.[28]

As the 1878 directive indicated, "wayward children" who had been subject solely to parental authority in the Edo period now came under the jurisdiction of the police. The language used to describe the status of those considered mad and their confinement also shifted. Instead of *ranshinsha* to refer to a mad person, the term *fūtennin* was used. This term had first appeared in an official document in the *Shinritsu kōryō* of 1870, the Meiji penal code in place before what became known as the Old Criminal Code was instituted in 1882. If *ranshinsha* was a general word, the equivalent perhaps of "madman" or "madwoman," then *fūtennin* was a specialized term with legal and medical resonances, along the lines of "insane person" or "mental patient." Terms describing confinement changed, too. Phrases commonly used in the preceding era such as "placement in a cage" (*kan'nyū*) were replaced with "enchainment" (*sako*), and the location of the confinement began to be called "private residence" (*shitaku*) rather than the former "family residence" (*kataku*) in order to distinguish it from confinement in newly established public asylums and hospitals. The word "nursing or caregiving" (*kango,* 看護) was displaced by its homonym "custody" (*kango,* 監護) and the related term "confinement" (*kanchi,* 監置). The police ordinance framed the work of the family as custody, emphasizing legal protective care or guardianship as opposed to everyday caregiving.

Prefectures quickly followed suit, issuing their own ordinances governing the mentally ill. Although the ordinances varied among prefectures, many specified in detail the administrative procedures and material requirements of home confinement.[29] Chiba prefecture issued "Regulations for the Management of Insane Persons (*fūtennin*)" in 1889, a thirteen-article ordinance that declared it essential that all "insane persons," regardless of whether they were confined or not, register with the police and be accompanied in all public places by a designated legal guardian. Hygienic standards were imposed, dictating how much sunlight and air circulation the "enchainment room" ought to receive. The use of forceful restraints, whether iron chains or ropes, was prohibited, as was the placement of flammable materials near the room. Families were subject to fines if they did not follow the terms of the ordinance.[30] Although the content of the various prefectural ordinances was more or less the same, the language used to describe the mentally unsound person or the practice of home confinement, as well as the procedure of attaining permission for either home or institutional confinement, was not uniform. Only with the passage of a national law was a measure of uniformity achieved.

The first national law concerning those considered mad was passed in 1900. Known as the Custody Law for the Mentally Ill (Seishinbyōsha kangohō; hereafter the Custody Law), it standardized the official language used to designate those considered mad and their confinement across various legal codes.[31] Consider the creation of the figure of the legal custodian (*kango gimusha*), one of the most significant changes to customary practice in the Custody Law. The newly created figure of the legal custodian shifted the locus of decision-making power for cases of confinement from the family–household association–village nexus of the preceding centuries to an individual within the family. The law required that each mentally ill person be assigned a custodian, usually the household head, who assumed all legal responsibility for the "patient." Whereas in the Edo period any member of the family could petition local authorities for confinement or release, the Custody Law allowed only the legal custodian to authorize confinement, whether at home in a cage-like enclosure or in one of the newly built public or private asylums. If a competent custodian could not be found, the city or prefectural administrative head would serve as the acting custodian. The Custody Law described in painstaking detail the qualifications and duties of the custodian—who could be a custodian, how a custodian reported to local authorities, where a custodian could confine his charge, and how a custodian would be punished for wrongful confinement.[32]

The figure of the legal custodian in the Custody Law of 1900 must be understood within the context of the late nineteenth-century creation of what many refer to as Japan's "family system." Beginning in the early 1870s, the Meiji state created a nationwide system of family registers, which recorded every individual in the country as a member of a household under the control of a male "household head," regardless of where he or she lived. As Sheldon Garon has pointed out, the Meiji regime "went much further than Tokugawa-era officials" of previous centuries, who had also used the family as "the first line of defence against poverty" and other social welfare needs "[but] had lacked the means to force families to care for destitute members whose kinship ties were dubious or who had left their native villages."[33] Under the Meiji system of family registers, combined with new public assistance laws, the state tracked down individual relatives recorded in the registers and ordered them to provide assistance to needy kin.

The Civil Code of 1898 further reinforced such notions of familial responsibility. The Civil Code was a collection of private laws that pertained to the relationships between individuals, as opposed to public laws that addressed the relationships between the state and individuals or organizations. Civil law had existed for centuries, but the laws were neither codified nor written until the Meiji period.[34] As part of a broader effort to repeal the "unequal treaties" signed in 1858 with the United States, Great Britain, the Netherlands, Russia, and France, Meiji leaders sought to create a legal system that would assure foreign powers of the legitimacy and reliability of local courts, as well as civil and criminal codes.[35] This primarily entailed creating a central judicial system and codifying law into written statues. In order to transform customary law into written statutes, Meiji legal reformers and scholars drew on the examples from France and Germany. The first draft of the Civil Code in 1890, later known as the Old Civil Code, was based on the Code Napoleon. But conservative critics claimed the 1890 version emphasized individual rights at the expense of undermining a "family system" that they considered the backbone of the Japanese polity and society. The title of a famous article written in 1891 by the legal scholar Hozumi Yatsuka captured this view: "The Civil Code Appears, and Loyalty and Filial Piety Disappear" (*Minpō idete, chūkō horobu*). Hozumi and others, including his brother and fellow legal scholar Hozumi Nobushige, were alarmed that, in the waning years of the nineteenth century, "the individual had begun to take the place of the family as the unit of society."[36] Hozumi Yatsuka offered a solution: give the household precedence over the individual by creating a legal foundation for the *ie* system of the Edo period, as newly imagined by Hozumi and his supporters. He especially advocated continuing the strong patriarchal authority and practice of primogeniture that had long characterized many samurai households. Ironically, Hozumi and other Meiji ideologues were trying to install a samurai model of family at a time when samurai status had been abolished.

The result was the revised Civil Code of 1898, which established the household or family (*ie*), rather than the individual, as the key unit of civil law. The patriarch, or household head (*koshu*), wielded great power over subordinate members, including his wife and children. He alone managed the family property, determined the disposition of family assets, chose the family's place of residence, and approved or disallowed marriages and adoptions of his children. The position of the household head would pass to the eldest son except in extraordinary circumstances. As Garon has shown, the revised Civil Code also required households to support their needy members, "establish[ing] an elaborate hierarchy of relationships that obligated the spouse, children and grandchildren, parents and grandparents, and then in-laws and siblings, reaching down to fairly distant relatives." The Civil Code of 1898, in other words, granted the state "the explicit legal authority to make the household the basis of welfare."[37]

The creators of the Custody Law for the Mentally Ill aimed to align its terms with those of the Civil Code of 1898 through the figure of the legal custodian. Ume Kenjirō, one of the three key jurists who revised the Civil Code, was the first to call for the creation of the Custody Law for the Mentally Ill. He and other jurists were primarily concerned that the Civil Code achieve comprehensive coverage and remain consistent with other legal statutes.[38] Ume thereby appealed to the Home Ministry to create a supplemental law concerning the mentally ill. In September 1899, the Home Ministry requested that the Central Committee on Hygiene (Chūō eiseikai) introduce such legislation:

> Although the Civil Code addresses the protection of insane persons (*fūtennin*), it is limited to the protection of such persons' property and does not cover the protection of their body and rights, as well as the effect that the insane have on the peace and order (*chian*) of society. Thus, the reason for proposing this bill is to acknowledge the necessity to establish a law concerning the control (*torishimari*) of the mentally ill at the administrative level.[39]

Jurists and bureaucrats within the Home Ministry framed their request for a law concerning "insane persons" as a two-pronged call for protections: the protection of the "body and rights" of afflicted individuals but that of others in society "peace and order," too. To achieve both forms of protection, the Custody Law replicated the logic of the Civil Code, subsuming individual rights under the concept of custodianship. In what amounted to a reinforcement of the idea that the household was the primary unit of society, mentally ill people were placed under the care of individual custodians in their families.

Technically, the Custody Law allowed for a range of persons to serve as legal custodian. Article 1 stated that "a guardian (*kōkennin*), spouse, relative to the fourth degree, or head of household shall take on the duty of [custody] (*kango*) for a mentally ill person."[40] The term "guardian" alluded to a passage in the Civil Code that described how a case for "guardianship" arose "when a person of full age was adjudged incompetent (*kinjisan*)" because he was of "unsound mind" (*shinshin sōshitsu no jōtai*). A spouse, relative, household head, or even public procurator could become a "guardian," resulting in a broad range of people who could rightfully assume the role of a legal guardian for an individual deemed mentally ill. But in most cases, the household head was assumed to possess the greatest authority. As Kubota Seitarō of the Home Ministry argued during a special committee discussion in February 1900, "It is the general custom [in our country] for the figure of the household head to take care of the family, so even among those designated as a spouse, it is appropriate for a husband to [be a guardian] for his wife, but it has become increasingly said that it is inappropriate for a wife to be the legal custodian in charge of confinement."[41] Kubota predicted that the custodian of mentally ill persons would typically be the male patriarch of the family.[42] Until 1900, entire families with their neighbors and even village representatives had signed petitions for the confinement of the mentally ill. The 1900 Custody Law dictated thereafter that only the custodian, usually the male household head, was legally allowed to sign such documents, confine the ill, and serve as the contact person for local officials.

The Custody Law reinforced the family ideology enshrined in the Civil Code, namely the unquestionable authority of the patriarch and the social function of the family. Since the 1890s, Meiji ideologues allied with the state had sought to construct the family as the moral foundation of the nation at a time of social and ideological crisis. As Ken Ito has summarized, if the late nineteenth century had ushered in "the social dislocations attendant upon industrialization and urbanization, as well as the ideological challenges posed by such new concepts as popular rights, individualism, and socialism, then the 'traditional' family could be used as a force for order, an institution for the proper location and training of citizens within the national hierarchy."[43] This ideology helped justify the state's reliance on the family as the primary provider of social welfare, whether for those considered mad, ill, or indigent. At the same time, the Custody Law pointed to the risks of relying on families, since they would at times resort to confinement under dubious circumstances. Over half the articles in the Custody Law thus explained the fines and punishments for wrongful confinement, that is, confinement without the approval of local authorities or with falsified documents. Submitting a falsified report could land a custodian in jail for up to one year. Doctors who falsified diagnosis forms were subject to similar penalties.

Although the passage of a law that regulated confinement on a national level was unprecedented, it did not significantly change families' actual practices of confinement. Of course, the new regulations detailed in the Custody Law, which influenced revisions to prefectural laws concerning the mentally ill, were bureaucratic matters that required attention. Families were compelled to learn new bureaucratic vocabularies of madness and care when filing paperwork for permission to use a confinement room. They encountered such new psychiatric terms as "mentally ill person" (*seishinbyōsha*) instead of older and more colloquial terms like "mad person" (*ranshinsha*) and such legalistic phrases as "private [residential] confinement" (*shitaku kanchi*) as opposed to references to "cages" (*ori*) and "parlor prisons" (*zashikirō*). Families and local officials alike learned these new vocabularies at the same time, as suggested by a publication in 1904 entitled "A Record of Questions and Answers about the Custody Law."[44] Intended for consultation by police and other local officials, the publication answered basic questions about the law, defined new terminology, and provided templates of forms both for families requesting permission to confine and for officials deciding whether to grant or deny permission.

Still, the impact of the Custody Law on actual practice remained limited partly because prefectural ordinances—and not the new national law—continued to determine the specific terms of both "private confinement" (*shitaku kanchi*) in homes and public confinement sponsored by local officials, usually in public-run detention centers, hospitals, or even the residences of other people.[45] The Custody Law did not even aim to encourage or enforce confinement in homes or hospitals. In fact, it made confinement more difficult by penalizing improper detention and setting standards for home custody. Its purpose was to regulate rather than to promote the centuries-old custom of confinement. For their part, families continued to use home confinement because of the social pressures exerted by a long-standing "culture of domestic responsibility," which held families morally responsible for the criminal and socially disruptive acts of its members.[46] With few other options on hand, families, particularly those in rural areas, resorted to confining members who were afflicted by madness that made them prone to violence. Under such constraints, the regulations detailed in the Custody Law, as well as their ideological valences, had minimal effect on everyday life, where it did not always matter whether the legal custodian was the male household head of the family, for instance, since the bulk of the daily physical and emotional labor of care fell on the shoulders of women.

Women's Labor of Care in the Making of Family

Women's physical and emotional caregiving labor within families enabled the practice of home confinement. Without women's labor, there would have been no one to tend to the bathing, toileting, and nourishing of the confined person. Without women's labor, many of the confined would not have survived. This is not to say that men and children did not partake in the care and custody of mentally disturbed members; confinement affected everyone living under the same roof. But women were expected to engage in the mundane and arduous tasks of caring for incapacitated members to a much greater extent than men in the family were. Also, the majority of confined individuals were men, so it often fell to the women in the family to navigate the complex bureaucratic process of obtaining permission to confine or release afflicted members, as well as make decisions about treatment and care. Without women's mental, emotional, and physical labor, the very "family" on which the state relied to provide for incapacitated and sick members would not have existed. Not a single observer of home confinement at the turn of the twentieth century commented on this gendered domestic economy of care that made home confinement possible in the first place. State and medical authorities documenting the practice across the country, as well as affected families themselves, took women's labor for granted.

Women's caregiving labor is mentioned throughout records of home confinement, including psychiatrist Kure Shūzō and medical student Kashida Gorō's report published in 1918, "Actual Conditions of Home Confinement and Statistical Observations of the Mentally Ill" (*Seishinbyōsha shitaku kanchi no jikkyō oyobi sono tōkeiteki kansatsu*). From 1910 to 1916, Kure Shūzō, the head of the Department of Psychiatry at Tokyo Imperial University's medical school, led a team of twelve psychiatrists in collecting information, statistics, floor plans, and photographs of home confinement in fifteen prefectures, most clustered near Tokyo, but some as far as Hiroshima in the southwest and Aomori in the northeast. In 1918, Kure and Kashida selected over 100 among the 364 observed cases and published their official report in the esteemed *Tokyo Journal of Medical Science* (*Tōkyō igakukai zasshi*).[47] Each case that appeared in the report offered information about the family's treatment of the mentally ill person, from the number of times the afflicted member was bathed each week to the types of food served to him or her throughout the day. The report is sprinkled with descriptions of women performing a range of domestic work for their confined husbands, sons, daughters, mothers, cousin, and in-laws. Much of the work involved the usual laundering, sewing, and cooking that they were expected to perform anyway. As the report reveals, women changed mosquito netting in the summer, swept floors, and passed meals through the bars of confinement rooms two or three times a day.[48]

Some daily tasks, such as cleaning and bathing, became much harder when performed for a mentally afflicted member. Items would be dirtied again within hours or a day or two because many of the confined ripped and soiled their clothing and bedding. In fact, many of the individuals surveyed by the psychiatrists suffered from conditions that made them prone to handling and smearing their own feces on their clothes, bedding, and walls. In the case of confined women, their clothing and bedding were often stained with menstrual blood. The stench of waste matter and blood filled many rooms. Bathing, too, required intensive labor on the part of family members, with some even calling on the police for help. In order to bathe the person, families used a bathtub in the house, prepared a separate tub, or visited a public bath. The arms and legs of agitated and quiet individuals alike were tied during baths for fear of resistance that might endanger either the afflicted person or the caretaker. In many cases families stopped bathing them altogether because of the difficulties involved.

When families unraveled in the face of madness, women stepped in to try to stitch together the fraying edges of kinship. In records from Ōita prefecture, for instance, an older sister of an afflicted woman served as the designated legal custodian and presented a narrative of suffering in the paperwork she submitted to gain permission to confine. Her younger sister had given birth to her third child in 1938, but soon thereafter drowned this daughter in a nearby well. There is no explanation for this drowning in the documentation, other than a brief comment that the birth mother was unwell. At first she was simply registered at the local police office as a mentally disturbed but unconfined person. But her condition quickly worsened. She became verbally and physically aggressive, throwing bowls of food at her sister, brother-in-law, and female servant during meals and yelling at them to "get out." During prolonged "fits" (*hossa*), the woman could not recognize anyone or anything around her. Once confined, the older sister seems to have regularly tended to the woman with relatively more consideration than in other cases, though it is possible that the sister was simply more meticulous about recording details regarding meal plans and activities in documents submitted to local prefectural authorities. Still, the degree of detail suggests that the woman's older sister felt compelled to demonstrate the care being provided, especially her adherence to hygienic standards, which she may have known was expected by local authorities. The sister explained that she and others regularly bathed the confined woman and cleaned her bedding and clothes, as well as brushing her hair and even applying makeup on days when "she was in a good mood."[49]

Women's work may not be hidden in the historical archive, but it is rendered invisible when the word "family" is substituted for "women." "Family" stood in for "women" in descriptions of those who performed the caregiving labor required to sustain home confinement. Common were such observations as "the patient's family did not have much flexibility in their lifestyle and so the caretaking was insufficient, as they must devote all their time to silk work."[50] Silk work had long been almost exclusively women's work, with men only cultivating the mulberry trees whose leaves were fed to silkworms and women responsible for raising the silkworms, reeling thread from the cocoons, and weaving silk cloth.[51] To say that "the patient's family" did not have the time to properly take care of its confined member because "they must devote all their time to silk work" meant more precisely that the women in the family were too overwhelmed by the demands of silk work to be able to provide sufficient care to the "patient." The substitution of "family" for "women" in this case does not deny the reality of a gendered economy of care within the household, but signals that those bearing witness to home confinement considered the substitution natural and unproblematic. Such an obvious facet of family life hardly merited comment.

At times, the expectation that women perform the labor of cleaning and care reached extremes. Mentally disturbed women, for instance, were sometimes expected to care for themselves. A confined woman observed by psychiatrist Kimura Onari in 1911, whose husband "led the life of a ruffian," had been confined by her husband and his mistress.[52] When she showed signs of an "illness" and became violent, her husband, his mistress, and his younger brother rolled her into a *futon* or thick bedding for five days. Although she was pregnant at the time, they proceeded to strip her naked and tie an iron chain around her abdomen, fastening it to a nearby wall with a padlock. Kimura took note of the scars that remained on her belly. After being in chains for twelve days, she was then moved to her confinement room, a subsection of the grain storage shed. She was occasionally provided with food and was washed once or twice a year, but she was expected to clean the confinement room and tend to herself in nearly all other ways. If no close female kin lived with or nearby a confined woman, the latter was often neglected to the point of starvation and death. A forty-one-year-old woman in Yamanashi prefecture became mentally disturbed after the death of her husband left her and her children deeply impoverished. In 1911, psychiatrist Saitō Tamao found her emaciated, under-dressed, and unclean in a dilapidated cage-like room. The room appeared to have no opening as an entrance or exit. Although the woman's adolescent son was her legal guardian, she was supported by her male cousin, who stopped by occasionally on his way back home from the fields. When asked about his female cousin's condition, he replied with only curses. The psychiatrist wrote in his report that "it seems [the male cousin] wishes for the woman's speedy death." Nothing in Saitō's report suggested the presence of a female caretaker.

Nor were elderly women exempt from the labor of caregiving. Often weakened themselves by age and sickness, elderly mothers took responsibility for caring for their adult sons. One mother in Nagano tended to her son in confinement as both his legal guardian and daily caregiver. Her son, a former soldier, showed signs of what was euphemistically called by psychiatrists "unclean behavior" (*fuketsu kōi*), or the touching and smearing of excrement. His

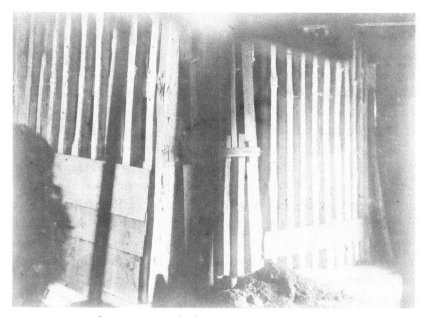

FIGURE 2.1 Confinement room of a forty-one-year-old woman in Yamanashi prefecture, c. 1911. Photograph courtesy of the Komine Institute.

mother did not have the strength to do more than give him three meals a day. Twice a month she hired a laborer to bathe him and clean the room.[53] Sisters and sisters-in-law were also commonly called upon as caretakers. A confined man in the same prefecture of Nagano, who had been confined for hitting his family members, was taken care of by his brother's wife, who left his soiled clothing and quilt out to dry during the day and returned it to the room at night.[54] And a woman confined for wandering the streets of Nagano after her divorce was in the custody of her brother-in-law, but her younger sister provided most of her care, cleaning the room three times a month.[55]

Women performed the bulk of the labor of caregiving, but were still expected to tend to the productive or farm-oriented labor of the household as well. Women in rural farm households did not stop working "outside" the home in the early twentieth century, even as urban-centric middle-class ideologies promoted ideas about women limiting their role to the domestic sphere. Rural women continued to spend time cultivating fields, harvesting silkworms, sunning grain, and pounding millet. But men increasingly performed less reproductive labor—childrearing, shopping, cleaning, cooking, and more—than in the preceding era, increasingly focusing on cultivating fields and other farm work. Women were thus generally expected to bear the burden of both the labor of farm work and the labor of care. Most families needed all able-bodied members to help with the farm work and could not afford to lose many laboring hands to the supervision of the confined. Many psychiatrists who surveyed cases of home confinement in the early twentieth century mentioned how the demands of farm work constrained the ability of "families" to look after their afflicted member, suggesting that women were overburdened.[56]

Psychiatrists like Kure Shūzō, the lead author of the 1918 report, criticized the additional caretaking work that was forced upon families.[57] Kure bemoaned the extreme neglect of the confined. "It is not possible," he wrote, "to suppress our sympathy for the [misfortune]" in such dire conditions. "However, we do not think families give this kind of thoughtless and cruel treatment intentionally. It is not that [persons interacting with the patient] have no sympathy or compassion. They are, after all, relations of parents and children, siblings, and couples."[58] In Kure's view, families neglected the mentally ill not out of cruelty, but because the demands of farm work prevented them from providing proper care. He added that many of the already-poor families were reduced to extreme poverty when forced to look after the sick. Kure thus did not blame the families for the miseries of home confinement, but he was convinced that families were ill equipped to be caretakers. They did not, he said, have the experience of taking care of patients with dementia who engaged in "unclean behavior." "We must think about how, in the face of such illnesses, families that have no experience in giving care have no idea what to do. [Overwhelmed] with hardship and worry (*shinrō*), in the end such [dire] conditions result."[59] Although entire families were affected by the double demands of caregiving and farm work, women faced a particularly heavy burden. Kure may have referred to "families" lacking the skills, knowledge, and wherewithal to care for the confined, but he could just as easily have specified that women in families were the ones "[overwhelmed] with hardship and worry" as they struggled in the face of having "no idea what to do."

Variations on the expression "no idea what to do" appear in records and reports of home confinement, at times directly from interviewed family members and at others from observing psychiatrists. The expression certainly captures what psychiatrists like Kure referred to as the hopelessness and helplessness that families faced. But it also evokes the tremendous efforts that women and families exerted to try to stitch back together life itself, "often with coarse thread," to echo anthropologist Sarah Pinto.[60] Such efforts involved grappling with profound ambiguities and paradoxes. Confinement was a practice that existed in the spaces between protection and punishment, for instance. It primarily served to protect those who lived with and among a mentally unstable person who was prone to violence. According to the Kure report, 112 out of 405 listed reasons for home confinement were related to such violence as throwing items, hitting family members, shouting threats, and breaking household objects.[61] Restricting the afflicted person's movements kept other family members safe. It was also common for families to choose to confine members because the latter wandered the village and mountains.[62] But more so than fear for the safety and well-being of the wandering person, it was the possibility of him or her committing crime or other socially unacceptable behavior that promoted families to lock him or her up. Mentally disturbed members were thus confined for fear of both actual and potential antisocial acts. The physical and bodily restraint of mentally afflicted members was meant to enable the freedom of mind and movement of others in the family. Yet such freedom came with caveats and constraints. Whether confined or not, the work of caring for a mentally disturbed person taxed women and families to the point that at times they must have felt that they, too, were living in cages.

The psychiatric archive of home confinement obscures some of the emotional and moral ambiguities and contradictions of living with confinement because psychiatrists aimed to present clear evaluations and classifications of the practice. For instance, psychiatrists categorized observed cases as "good," "bad," and "extremely bad," using hygienic conditions as their main metric. They assessed the quality of care and caregivers in similar terms. In the case of the family whose story opened this chapter, the observing psychiatrists criticized the wife and mother of the confined man and son for being "abusive" and "lazy," especially considering that they were a relatively affluent family who could afford to provide better care. But in a segment of reported speech, the report provides a glimpse of the wife's experience: she "simply did not know what else to do" besides confine and restrain her husband and son once they began showing signs of violence and "unclean behavior."[63] Even for relatively affluent rural families, alternatives to home confinement were limited. New psychiatric hospitals tended to be built in cities, and even then confinement in a hospital was not necessarily seen as a desirable and viable alternative to keeping the afflicted at home.

As much as women and families felt trapped by the lack of alternatives to home confinement, they tended to the tasks of daily living in an effort to hold together the material, physical, and emotional ties and obligations of family. Both literally and figuratively, caregiving labor tied together the people and spaces of the home and neighborhood. Although cage-like rooms signaled the exclusion and separation of a member from their family and surroundings, confinement rooms were embedded in the domestic and social spaces of the house and village, and women caregivers moved from one space to another in the course of the day. Most confinement rooms were built either inside a bedroom or storeroom inside the main house. Fewer were built as attachments to the main house, and even fewer were built as separate structures or makeshift edifices connected to sheds in the yard or storehouses near the farm.[64] The tendency to build confinement cages in heavily trafficked areas of the home and farm suggests that caregiving for the confined person was integrated into the daily rhythms of both reproductive and productive labor on the farm. Confining a person inside a storehouse was not necessarily a sign of neglect. Some families certainly showed little regard for the well-being of individuals confined in such places, but storehouses were generally considered the most valuable and protected structure of the farmhouse, since the foodstuffs stockpiled there were sources of income and sustenance for families. Tending to the people and items housed in a storehouse constituted attempts to sustain lives and livelihoods.

Daily caregiving labor built and rebuilt worlds that imploded when a family member was locked up in a cage inside their own home. Women's labor sustained families afflicted by madness, but the same labor also sapped their strength and will. Focusing on this feminized caregiving labor reveals ways in which the ties of family were contingent on domestic acts of labor usually perceived as ordinary and minor. Contrary to what Meiji ideologues and lawmakers touted about the unchanging, stable, and natural Japanese family, women's caregiving labor exposes the fragility of "family."

Most families did not qualify for the little public assistance that was available, but under exceptional circumstances local officials stepped in as substitute guardians. One such circumstance involved families that were extremely impoverished. Local officials first assessed the family's finances and searched for the existence of other relatives and kin. If the family qualified, village heads and other local figures served as de facto legal guardians and drew on prefectural funds to confine the afflicted individual in a hospital, local facility, or private residence.[65] State officials also intervened in cases where mentally disturbed individuals found wandering the streets could not recall their names, addresses, or any other identifying marker. When a police officer found a woman believed to be in her early thirties wandering in the streets of Takasaki City in Gunma prefecture in 1910, he took her to an accommodation for "transient sick people." She was soon registered as a ward of

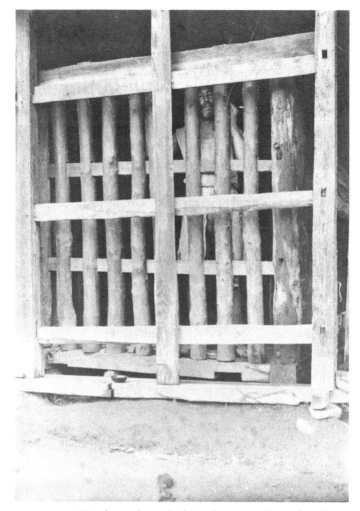

FIGURE 2.2 Wooden enclosure built inside main residence for a thirty-eight-year-old farmer in Gunma prefecture, c. 1910. Photograph courtesy of the Komine Institute.

the prefectural governor as well as that of the mayor of Takasaki.[66] A national law in 1899 required prefectures to build such shelters for "sick wanderers" (*kōrobyōsha*), and some eventually dedicated some rooms to those considered mentally ill. The Isei Sanatorium in Kōfu City in Yamanashi prefecture, for instance, reserved one room for those under "public confinement" under the terms of the Custody Law of 1900. When psychiatrist Saitō Tamao visited the sanatorium, he noted that a hired caretaker (*kanrisha*) supervised some light work performed by "patients" who were not too sick to work. Saitō praised

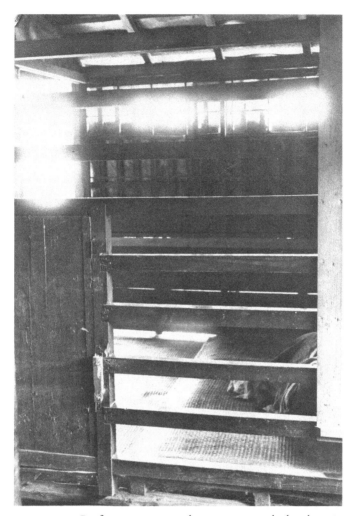

FIGURE 2.3 Confinement room inside a structure attached to the main residence in Gunma prefecture, c. 1910. The forty-two-year-old woman had been confined in the room for twelve years at the time of observation. Photograph courtesy of the Komine Institute.

the caretaker and the facility for implementing a "family-like approach to care (*kazokuteki kangohō*).[67]

Such cases of public confinement often relied on the labor of women, too, usually as hired help.[68] A mentally disturbed man living in what was known as a "sick house for the poor" (*kyūryōbyōshitsu*) in a city in Chiba prefecture, for instance, was cared for by an elderly woman hired by the city. A psychiatrist who visited the facility remarked that he was impressed that the city had such

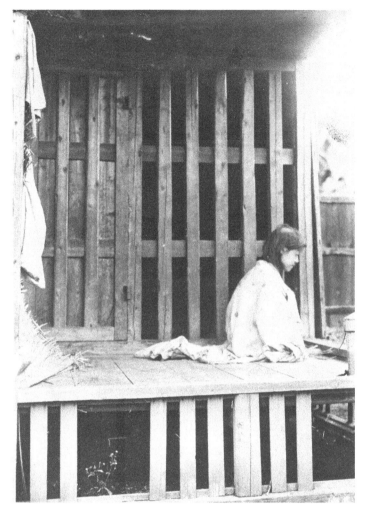

FIGURE 2.4 Mentally disturbed young woman found wandering in Takasaki City, Gunma prefecture. Placed in a public shelter for "sick wanderers." Photograph courtesy of the Komine Institute.

a public facility, but still lamented the inadequacy of the treatment and care. He criticized the hired elderly woman for lacking "the kindness that is needed when caring [for a patient]," pointing out that she herself was an impoverished person hired to do a job for which she had no specialized training.[69] In another instance, the headman of a village in Toyama prefecture served as the legal guardian of a man placed in publicly funded confinement, but hired the man's sixty-seven-year-old mother for 15 *sen* a day to tend to his daily needs. The man had started to show "signs of mental abnormality" after his wife,

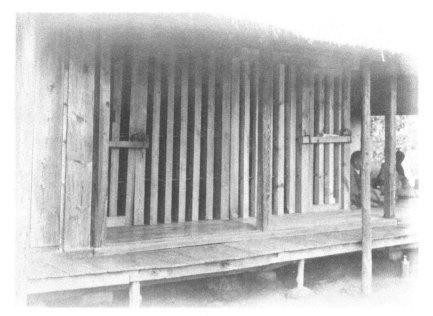

FIGURE 2.5 The Isei Sanatorium in Kōfu City, Yamanashi prefecture. One room was dedicated to the confinement of mentally disturbed city residents. Photograph courtesy of the Komine Institute.

unable to further endure their poverty, abandoned him and their children and ran away from home. When he began to suffer hallucinations and became violent toward himself and others, the village headman took charge of placing him in a confinement room built near the town's main office. His caretaker-mother lived only about 200 meters away in a rented room, tending to both him and his children.[70]

Women, whether hired or not, were not significantly relieved of their burdens with the passage of a new law in 1919 that ordered more public assistance for families coping with madness. The psychiatric campaign against home confinement helped pass the Mental Hospitals Law (*Seishinbyōin hō*), which called for the expansion of hospital-based public provisions for the mentally ill. As historian Akihito Suzuki has summarized, "the [Law] empowered the Minister of Home Affairs to order the prefectures to build public asylums in which poor patients were to be kept, and that half of the cost for building the hospital and one-sixth of the cost for maintaining the patients would be covered by the central government."[71] The Kure report contributed to this push for hospitalization, with Diet members discussing its findings and acknowledging the limited number of psychiatric facilities in

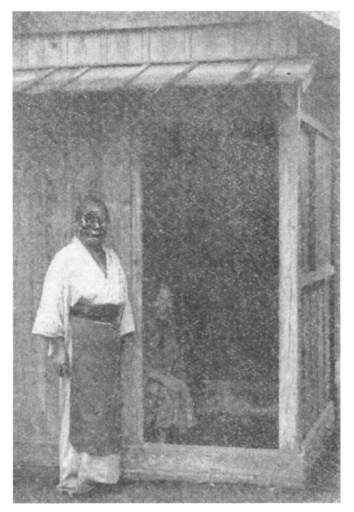

FIGURE 2.6 Elderly woman hired as caretaker of a mentally disturbed man residing in a public "sick house" in Chiba prefecture. Reproduced from Case 100, *SBSK*, 79.

the country. Minister of Home Affairs Tokonami Takejirō repeatedly cited the figure that only 4,000 out of 60,000 mental patients were confined in hospitals. This rate of confinement was far below "the western standard" and a "national shame."[72] Yet the passage of the Mental Hospitals Act did not create the nationwide system of hospital-based care that Kure and his fellow psychiatrists desired. Instead, along with the Custody Law of 1900, it helped create two distinct forms of caregiving in urban and rural areas, both of which were implicitly premised on women's caregiving labor.

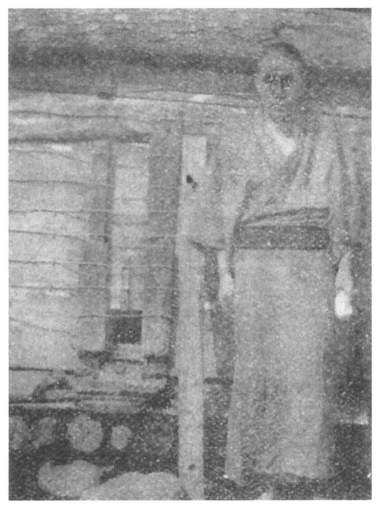

FIGURE 2.7 Sixty-seven-year-old mother hired as caretaker for her son in public confinement under the terms of the Custody Law of 1900 in Toyama prefecture. Reproduced from Case 102, *SBSK*, 81–82.

After the passage of the Mental Hospitals Act, rural families tended to continue to resort to home confinement, whereas those in urban areas sought alternative care in hospitals, for several reasons. Rural houses were more spacious than urban residences, allowing families to build cages inside rooms or as separate rooms attached to the main building. Making such structural changes to houses was easier for residents of rural towns and villages, more than 80 percent of whom owned their houses, whereas city dwellers lived in row houses (*nagaya*) and apartment-like units that were difficult to alter.[73]

More significant, there was a strong disincentive for public authorities in the countryside to pay for the establishment of public hospitals when families continued to bear the cost of managing the mentally ill under the terms of the Custody Law of 1900. By 1935, only twenty-two out of forty-seven prefectures had public psychiatric beds, most of which were located in private hospitals rather than public asylums. Whereas cities like Tokyo and Osaka placed approximately half of all registered mentally ill individuals in hospitals, the rates of hospitalized patients in rural areas stayed below 1 percent, leading historian Akihito Suzuki to conclude that "[t]he Mental Hospitals Act achieved virtually nothing in rural areas."[74] Some rural families sent mentally ill members to nearby temples and shrines for treatment, but these religious sites were small-scale businesses, each of which housed a small number of patients, usually no more than thirty. The religious sites were considered places of extended domestic care, rather than a stable and long-term alternative site of care outside the family home in rural areas.[75]

In contrast, urban areas witnessed the growth of psychiatric hospitals with the passage of the Mental Hospitals Act. Instead of building public mental hospitals, local authorities allowed private psychiatric facilities to allot a certain number of beds for patients whose treatments and care were paid by the local government. As a result, public psychiatric provision relied upon the private sector. "Whether a prefecture could have public psychiatric beds," as Suzuki writes, "depended directly on the feasibility of running a private hospital there. One needed a substantial number of relatively wealthy families who would pay for psychiatric services in order to build psychiatric provision for poor lunatics."[76] Since the necessary critical mass of wealthy clients was concentrated in cities, most rural areas were left without psychiatric hospitals.

Families often formed networks that stretched across urban and rural areas, using both home confinement and hospitalization to accommodate mentally ill members.[77] Rural families with sufficient financial resources sent mentally ill members to hospitals in cities, and urban families sent back mentally ill members to their parental homes in the countryside. A woman from Mie prefecture, about 200 miles west of Tokyo, moved to the city to live with her husband and his parents. In 1911, she showed signs of mental illness, which her husband attributed to the mental exhaustion she experienced while nursing [taking care of] her father-in-law at home. Although the couple moved out of the husband's parents' house, the woman's condition continued to deteriorate. On one occasion she claimed to be an empress and on another she tried to hang herself. After two stays in two different psychiatric hospitals in Tokyo, she was sent back to her parental home in the countryside of Mie.

In November 1913, she was returned to Tokyo and admitted to the Ōji Brain Hospital for three weeks. In another case, a man from Gunma prefecture who moved to Tokyo with his wife and children was diagnosed with neurasthenia in 1928. When his condition worsened, his wife and children were sent back to her parental family in Gunma and the man's older brother moved with his family from Gunma to Tokyo to take care of him. The couple divorced three years later, and the man was incorporated into his brother's household as a dependent member. His sister-in-law tended to his daily needs but he proved difficult to care for, refusing to eat food prepared by her, becoming violent when refused pocket money, and wandering the streets. After seven years of care at home, he was hospitalized.[78] In both cases, mental illness was managed through family networks, but proved disruptive to families, temporarily and legally breaking up households for the purpose of care. The establishment of hospitals hardly removed the family as the primary agent of care in the management of the mentally disturbed. Instead, the work of families, and especially the women therein, intensified and broadened across the urban and rural divide well into the twentieth century.

From its origins in the Edo period until the twentieth century, home confinement persisted as a common means of managing mentally disturbed family members who were prone to violence, especially for those living in rural areas. Faced with few other options, families made the difficult decision to restrict the movements of their disturbed family member in storage sheds and cage-like structures. The Edo-period association of such confinement to moral and physical rehabilitation, as when used with disobedient sons, endured into the early twentieth century, with some families desperately hoping that the passage of time within such a place might somehow restore health. Yet few confined persons recuperated under confinement; the majority experienced further deterioration of their mental and physical health.

Although the psychiatrists who left behind visual and textual records of home confinement emphasized the neglect, abuse, and cruelty of the practice, focusing on the women who performed most of the daily caregiving labor underscores their intense efforts to sustain the lives and dignity of their relatives. Women not only shouldered the day-to-day emotional and physical labor involved in the care of the confined person, but had to navigate new legal regulations and bureaucratic processes established by the local police and prefectural authorities to do so.[79] They provided food, cleaned the room, and laundered bedding and clothes, while usually watching their confined family member's condition deteriorate. Women's domestic caregiving labor for the confined makes it possible to see not only how "care" is often indistinguishable from neglect and abandonment, but also its lethality—the way it can psychologically damage and physically deplete those compelled to provide it. This labor enacted kinship, too: it repeatedly performed, instantiated, and questioned what officials, ideologues, and others were touting as effortlessly natural. Even once sites of care began to proliferate outside the home in the early twentieth century, with psychiatric hospitals, clinics, and rest homes made available to those who could financially afford them, "family" remained central to ways of caring for and understanding forms of mental and emotional affliction, especially for women. When the women who labored to provide care fell ill, they turned, for better or worse, to the domain and language of kinship.

3

Hysteria in the Marketplace

ON OCTOBER 10, 1919, the *Yomiuri* newspaper printed a nineteen-year-old woman's anonymous submission to a column called "Consultations on Home Hygiene." "I am troubled these days," she wrote, "because the most trivial things bother me. I am unhappy due to ceaseless mental and emotional fatigue (*kokoro ga kizukare*)," all the more alarming to her because she was soon to be married. After mentioning that her physical health seemed fine, with the exception that she was losing weight and would like to regain it, she implored the doctor to explain "how to cure [this condition], what medicine to take." The consulting doctor Okada Michikazu responded with a clear diagnosis: "Your illness (*byōki*) is likely hysteria." After establishing that this illness was common among women, he described hysteria simply as what had long been commonly known as the "path of blood" (*chi no michi*) or "pain flowing from the heart-spirit [vital energy]" (*ki kara yamai ga deru*). The most effective therapy, the doctor explained, included exercising, rubbing oneself with a cold wet towel every morning, minimizing idle thought, and going to sleep at an early hour. In terms of medication, he recommended taking sodium bromide under a doctor's supervision. As for her impending marriage, the doctor assured her that there was no cause for worry, for marriage would improve her mood (*kibun*) and restore her physical health.

This exchange between an anonymous young woman and male doctor in the pages of a national newspaper offers a glimpse into the "domestication" of hysteria in Japan at the turn of the twentieth century. "Domestication" entailed two interlinked processes: first, the translation and adaptation of a European medical diagnosis in Japanese popular discourse, and second, the creation of a seemingly natural link between "hysteria" and women's domestic lives. At first glance, these two processes of "domestication" might seem to signal a structural shift from home-based confinement to commercialized care for those

Madness in the Family. H. Yumi Kim, Oxford University Press. © Oxford University Press 2022.
DOI: 10.1093/oso/9780197507353.003.0004

considered mentally and emotionally disturbed. "Domestication" occurred, after all, within an expanding commercial marketplace of print media, medicinal products, and therapeutic services offered at such new sites of care as hospitals and clinics in urban areas. But as the term "domestication" suggests, the intimate and complex domains of family and kinship continued to impinge upon and provide the setting in which ailments like hysteria gained traction in Japan.

A growing mass print media industry enabled the "domestication" of a European-derived ailment in a Japanese context. In 1774, physician Sugita Genpaku had introduced the concept of "nerves" by coining the Japanese word *shinkei*, a translation of the term "Zenuw" that appeared in Johann Kulmus's *Anatomische Tabellen* (1722). Decades later, physician Ogata Koan elaborated on the concept of nerves by introducing "hysteria" and "hypochondria" as types of neurological illnesses in his *Practical Instructions of Mr. Fu* (*Fushi keiken ikun*, 1842), a thirty-volume compendium based on a Dutch translation of a German manual of medical practice, which became an authoritative reference work on Western medicine. Diseases of the nerves, Koan wrote, "is called hypochondria in men and hysteria in women."[1] Although Japanese psychiatrists and other medical specialists diagnosed men with hysteria, it became predominantly associated with women in popular discourse at the turn of the twentieth century.[2] From the 1880s onward, journalists, drug manufacturers, doctors, and others who produced articles and advertisements for newspapers, monthly magazines, pamphlets, manuals, and books described "hysteria" as an updated version of an older form of women's psychosomatic affliction long known in Japan as "path of blood" (*chi no michi*). The same groups perpetuated the notion that women and men suffered from distinct forms of "nervous illness," with hysteria becoming the pejorative feminine counterpart of a more honorable form of masculine nervousness called "nerve fatigue" (*shinkei suijaku*), or neurasthenia.[3] While neurasthenic male intellectuals, students, and bureaucrats were exhausted by unrelenting economic competition and ideologies of success and striving, women became associated with a theatrical and dramatic excess of emotion in the form of hysteria.[4]

With the help of the mass print media, hysteria quickly evolved from medical jargon to household word. Mothers complained about their married daughters showing signs of *hisu*, the casual abbreviation for the condition. Men described their wives, older sisters, and aunts as having hysterical personalities that made the women susceptible to depression, anxiety, and excitability. Hysteria came to be so associated with women that psychiatrist

Sugie Tadasu complained in 1915 that it had become the default explanation for any kind of pain experienced by a woman, whether an injured foot or a mood fluctuation. Though perhaps exaggerated, Sugie's comment captures a sense of the ubiquity of hysteria as a catch-all term for women's disorders.

"Domestication" involved creating a seemingly natural link between hysteria and women's domestic and intimate familial lives, too. The concerns of the woman who wrote to *Yomiuri* newspaper about her marriageability were typical. Both she and Dr. Okada embedded her unease and suffering within the context of the pressure to marry and reproduce a family line. The woman was keenly aware of the implications of her condition for marriageability: women of her age were expected to be healthy in mind and body. The consulting doctor even suggests that the woman's impending marriage, which she declares is partly the source of her current anxiety, will in fact improve her mood and condition. He conflates cause and cure. Other doctors and commentators domesticated hysteria by designating women's hysteria as the source of crime and other transgressive behaviors, especially ones that violated the norms of the gender hierarchy and family expectations. They linked hysteria with women in a context of heightened anxieties about the viability of the "traditional" family, marriage, and conventional gender roles, as well as the perceived crisis of national decadence.[5]

Japanese diagnosticians and women embedded hysteria into a feminized domestic life at a time when sites of treatment outside the home began to proliferate, especially in urban areas. Between the mid-1910s and early 1930s, drug manufacturers, medical professionals, self-stylized healers, religious specialists, and other entrepreneurs helped extend sites of care for hysteria and other similar conditions from the home to an eclectic array of places. Enterprising physicians established private clinics and hospitals specializing in such areas as gynecology and hormone therapy. Mental healers founded local organizations that provided training in meditative and breathing techniques to help alleviate melancholy, headaches, and nervousness. Leaders of new religious groups offered counseling sessions for couples and groups. Even the police established personal consultation offices for women and men struggling with emotional and financial issues in the household. Unlike rural residents who remained limited to providing care and confinement in the home, urban consumers with some expendable income were able to lead what commonly became known as a "life of therapy" (*ryōhō seikatsu*) in search of remedies for their sufferings. A middle-class housewife in search of a cure for her nervous spasms might go from gynecologist to hypnotist in Tokyo, from a spiritual healer in the countryside to a shaman recommended by a friend.

Not all urban women were able to take advantage of the expansion of treatment possibilities outside the home. Women from less affluent families were disinclined to spend part of the household budget on medical treatment for themselves. They turned instead to purchasing cheaper herbal or patent medicines and relying on medical handbooks, home encyclopedias, newspaper articles, and women's magazine features offering advice to women about their bodily and mental afflictions.[6] The purchase of such new print media was, of course, a form of consumption and participation in a growing medical marketplace of media, goods, and services. Still, women other than those from the middle- and upper-classes residing in urban areas did not as readily consider using medical and therapeutic services offered outside the home. Nor did new services and sites of care provide a place for women that was entirely distinct and separate from their homes. Such new sites of care as psychiatric hospitals and therapy centers usually served as extensions of— rather than replacements for—home-based care.

Although women across classes subscribed to medical notions of feminine nervous illness that were embedded in domestic concerns such as marriage and family life, they rarely self-identified as hysterical in the way that many men labeled themselves as neurasthenic. In fact, many women either rejected or ignored the diagnosis of hysteria imposed on them by doctors, journalists, and family members, referring to their conditions with the generic term "illness" (*byōki*) and preferring to delve into the complexities of their domestic and psychological lives without using diagnostic labels. For many women, their illnesses occurred "off" their bodies and in the world of intimate relations of family.[7] They refused to localize their illness in their individual minds and bodies, invoking instead the influence of the relations of kin and family on their suffering. Women thus understood their illnesses in a family vernacular, a language that emphasized the interconnected nature of "body-selves" within kin networks. In managing their illnesses, many women had little recourse but to turn to the same family that they often saw as the source of suffering. Within families, women relied most heavily on their relationships with other women, from mothers to female cousins. Female sociality sustained but also attenuated familial ties as women coped with their mental and emotional afflictions.

Translating Hysteria in the Medical Marketplace

One of the first places where a Japanese reader would have come across hysteria in the late nineteenth century was print advertisements for mass-produced patent medicines (*baiyaku*). Beginning in the 1880s, advertisements for pills and elixirs claiming to ease the jittery nerves and mental exhaustion caused by nervous illnesses such as hysteria and neurasthenia began to appear in newspapers and magazines; on calendars and posters that decorated the walls of homes and retail shops; and on billboards, signposts, and telephone posts that lined the streets of towns, cities, and villages.[8] Propelled by the expansion of new print media and the replacement of woodblock printing with the printing press, advertisements for patent medicine saturated the print media to an unprecedented degree in the early twentieth century. In 1882, patent medicine advertisements occupied over 50 percent of the space in one national newspaper. In 1910 and onward, ads for patent medicine and cosmetics across fifty-seven newspapers outnumbered those for any other product, including books and magazines.[9] Among medicinal products to treat nervous illness, brand names like Chūjōtō ("Chūjō tonic"), Nōgan ("brain pills"), Kennōgan ("healthy brain pills"), and Shinseieki ("spirit relaxing elixir") crowded the pages of newspapers and magazines, many becoming standard products known throughout the country.

The proliferation of ads attests to the growth of the patent drug industry at a time when bodily health became central to politics and culture, making medicine a profitable business. Since the 1870s, the Meiji government had aimed to improve the health of its citizens by establishing a modern medical and public health system that could contend with epidemics of cholera and other acute infectious diseases introduced to Japan in the wake of the forced "opening" of treaty ports to Western imperialist powers. The state established new medical schools and a system of state licensing that elevated so-called Western medicine above such traditional or popular treatments as Chinese medicine, acupuncture, moxibustion, and massage. It created quarantine hospitals for sufferers of cholera, typhus, syphilis, and leprosy.[10] Government campaigns urged men and women to adopt new behaviors including drinking milk and using toothpaste, all for the sake of creating a large and healthy population capable of resisting Euro-American imperialism. As historian Susan Burns writes, "in the face of official and civil discourse that attacked patent medicines as at best useless and wasteful and at worst dangerous quackery that threatened public safety, manufacturers and advertisers sought to represent their products as an essential part of 'modern life' by linking them with technological advancement, the new ethos of nationalism, and the pleasures of bourgeois life."[11] Drug manufacturers such as Morita Jihei and Kishida Ginkō pioneered the development of marketing devices like illustrations, trademarks, slogans, and testimonials. These manufacturers yoked an emergent culture of mass consumption to national concerns about healthy minds and bodies to sell medicinal products.

"Hysteria" entered the commercial fray in the 1890s in advertisements for patent medicines that treated illnesses known in both medical and popular discourse as "women's disease" (*fujinbyō*). A term developed by Meiji gynecologists, sexologists, and hygienists, "women's disease" referred to a wide range of diseases that affected women, especially gynecological diseases such as venereal disease, infertility, and irregular menstruation, many of which supposedly had detrimental effects on sexual reproduction and the health of the fetus. Although such diseases had existed and been treated by physicians long before 1868, they took on new significance in the Meiji period as women's reproductive health came to be the object of investigation and classification by a state concerned with the overall health and strength of its population.[12] As young women were potential mothers who would bear and raise the nation's future citizens, their sexual health and reproductive physiology acquired national significance.

The category of "women's disease" pertained to the Meiji ideology of the "good wife, wise mother" (*ryōsai kenbo*). Deployed by the Education Ministry in 1898, "good wife, wise mother" became the slogan of the new nationwide network of girls' higher schools (*kōtō jogakkō*), a separate secondary education track for girls that would include moral education and homemaking skills, "channeling young women toward a domestic destiny rather than wage employment, cultural and intellectual pursuits, or political activities in the public sphere."[13] This new norm of womanhood required women to receive an adequate education so they could instruct their children and shape the next generation of citizens. The "good wife, wise mother" slogan became a central concept in the state's vision of womanhood from the late nineteenth century to the early 1930s, tested and modified by a range of people, including Ministry of Education officials, educators, intellectuals, journalists, feminists, and young women themselves. Few questioned the role of women to give birth to and raise children who would eventually fight, work, and reproduce for the sake of the nation. The health of women's reproductive bodies was thus central to official visions of motherhood.

But the path to motherhood was supposedly strewn with obstacles. Some argued that a woman's body, because its physiological complexity and constitutional weakness, might potentially prevent her from fulfilling her prescribed role as a "good wife, wise mother." Doctors who wrote about "women's disease" for the general public expressed concerns about such barriers. Sasaoka

Shōzō, for instance, wrote in the introduction to his *Instructions for Those with Women's Disease* (*Fujinbyōsha no kokoroe*, 1910):

> [W]omen get married, manage a household with their husbands, and raise healthy children in order to serve as the foundation for the flourishing of a family. They [also] serve as the foundation of a wealthy and powerful nation and ought to be the source of social harmony. Since they are entrusted with the highest of duties, they ought to maintain a body and [level of] wisdom that helps them carry out [this goal]. But compared to a man's body, a woman's body is weak and her reproductive organs are complicated, which significantly affects the functions of the entire body, and so it is more susceptible to disease. There are many cases of terrible illnesses of the uterus and related organs. As a result, women are unable to have children, bring weakness into the family, and lose a sense of enjoyment. The fact that there are many who cannot fulfill their duty as a woman is truly regrettable.[14]

Sasaoka's commentary exemplified the conservative outlook of many physicians promoting the interests not only of the state but also of their emerging professions. Specialists in women's disease would gain in prestige as more and more women sought their expertise. In their writings, they reduced the duty of women to domestic responsibilities toward husband and children and described women's bodies as either the savior or destroyer of familial and national health.

One such destructive malady was hysteria. The first signs of inclusion of hysteria into this mix of feminine ailments appeared in advertisements for patent drugs. Especially famous for the treatment of "women's disease" was the tonic known as Chūjōtō, an herbal concoction infused in hot water and consumed daily for the sake of promoting female reproductive health and easing the discomforts of menstruation, pregnancy, and childbirth. Released by the pharmaceutical company Tsushima Jutendō in 1893, Chūjōtō was among the most heavily advertised patent medicines on the market by the 1910s. A typical Chūjōtō advertisement spelled out the details of various women's ailments and their symptoms, which suggests that some of the diseases might have been unfamiliar to readers. Included in the list of women's ailments were "uterine disease" (*shikyūbyō*), irregular menstruation, frenzy (*nobose*), leucorrhea (vaginal discharge), and female nervousness, indicated variously by the terms "path of blood" (*chi no michi*), "hysteria" (*hisuterii*), and "women's nervousness" (*fujin shinkei*).

From the start, Chūjōtō advertisements introduced hysteria as an updated term for the condition long known in Japan as the "path of blood," a widely evoked phrase for feminine pains that appeared in early Japanese medical texts and literary works, a priest in 1362 being one of the first to write about the condition.[15] It was often associated with menopause in women as well as numerous nonspecific symptoms, including dizziness, palpitations, headaches, chilliness, stiff shoulders, and a dry mouth. The term itself implied the circulation of blood throughout the body, as well as its stoppages and overflows. But in the 1880s, as entries in popular medical encyclopedias and household manuals attest, the "path of blood" was elided with the new concept of hysteria. Matsumoto Ryōjun (Jun), physician to the last shogun and author of the medical handbook *Methods of Treatment for Various Diseases of the People* (*Minkan shobyō ryōchihō*, 1880), characterized the "path of blood" as a popularly known disease among women who exhibited mostly psychological symptoms such as depression, frenzy, and dizziness, recommending patent drugs like Sōshingan and Koshinen to help temper anger and dispel bad moods.[16] There was no mention of hysteria. By the 1890s, hysteria began to appear alongside the term "path of blood." In another one of his medical manuals, *Popular Medical Measures* (*Tsūzoku iryō benpō*, 1892), Matsumoto explained "path of blood" by emphasizing the fluctuation of moods and incorporating the term "hysteria":

> The path of blood, as it is popularly known, affects only women. The name of the illness is extremely vague, but in most cases, it is caused by a weakening of the brain [and nerves] and the head starts to hurt mostly in the area around the temples. The heart (*shinshin*) becomes depressed and [things] are not enjoyable. In extreme cases the [patient] cries or faints. . . . This illness occurs with uterine blood (*shikyūchi*) as well as young women's diseases (*shojobyō*). Not every case is one of real illness, but occurs when there is a momentary change in nerve functions, which is known as hysteria.[17]

Here, Matsumoto introduces hysteria as "a momentary change in nerve functions" that triggers the "path of blood," which in turn encompasses "a weakening of the brain," linking together in a generalized way Meiji neurological discourse with an older concept.

By enlisting hysteria as an updated word for "path of blood," patent drug advertisements helped bring the term into common parlance. The advertisements were instructive, informing consumers of changes in medical language and diagnoses. Yet the advertisers did not draw their notions of hysteria from medical textbooks aimed at doctors and other medical specialists. The earliest references to hysteria after 1868 in translations of American and European medical texts made no reference to possible Japanese counterparts to the disease.[18] Nor did patent drug advertisers adopt psychiatrist Kure Shūzō's "translation" of hysteria as "*zōsōbyō*" in his first major textbook of 1895, a diagnosis with ancient classical Chinese origins that would not have been well known among ordinary men and women.[19] They relied instead on the genre of popular medical handbooks, some written by licensed physicians like Matsumoto Jun, others by men with questionable qualifications who falsely attached the honorific title *hakase*, or doctor, to their names.

"Path of blood" and "hysteria" were not only represented as synonymous and interchangeable, but were often conflated with a third term, "female nervousness" (*fujin shinkei*). One advertisement for Chūjōtō in 1900 described those afflicted with "path of blood or hysteria" as "irritable, unable to sleep at night, worried about insignificant things, impatient, and short of breath."[20] Another in the same year, this time for a drug known as Shinseieki, explained the definition of hysteria as follows: "hysteria (*heesuterii*) [is] the generic term for women's disease (*fujinbyō*), nervous illness, path of blood (*chi no michi*), and persistently lingering illnesses (*burabura yamai*)."[21] Hysteria was presented as an all-encompassing term for these various ailments. The advertisement further clarified that "[hysteria] is the hypochondria (*hipokonderi*) of men," the female counterpart to a masculine form of nervousness that consumers presumably already knew about.

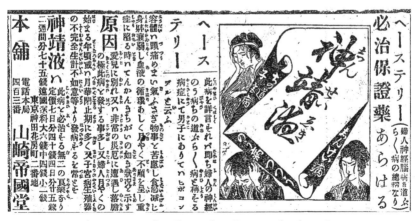

FIGURE 3.1 Advertisement for Shinseieki, *Yomiuri shimbun*, January 12, 1900. Reproduced by permission of Yamazaki Teikokudō Co., Ltd. and The Yomiuri Shimbun.

Advertisements for products like Chūjōtō offered visions of a future filled with domestic and reproductive bliss that aligned with official ideologies of gender and family. One of the most popular images was the figure of the healthy baby, poised high in the air in his father's outstretched arms, both parents lovingly gazing at the child. The advertisements often spoke of the challenges faced by couples who were unable to bear children and urged women to drink Chūjōtō to improve their chances of conception. The physical and emotional health of the woman, it was implied, determined the future of the family. In 1909 a drawing of an unusually brawny baby boy vigorously waving a carp streamer, his lips pressed in determination and his eyes looking into the distance, occupied the center of a newspaper advertisement.[22] He stands boldly, bursting forth from a gigantic fleshy peach. This is none other than an image of "Peach Boy," Momotarō, from the famous folktale of a boy born from a peach who, together with a dog, a monkey, and a pheasant, overcomes the monsters on Devil's Island, returning home laden with treasures. In an advertisement that detailed the symptoms of uterine and menstrual diseases, the image of the juicy and luscious peach from which the boy rises could not but evoke the idea of a "fruitful" vagina, seemingly cared for by treatment with Chūjōtō. Two vertically written slogans framed the right and left sides of the image of Momotarō: "A strong beloved child is born from a healthy woman" and "A healthy woman is produced by taking Chūjōtō."

Another common motif in Chūjōtō advertisements was the image of unhappy women, hair disheveled and sitting listlessly by themselves. In an ad from 1910, the viewer's eyes are drawn to the bottom-left corner in which a woman, a hand on her cheek, leans against an armrest.[23] She appears tired and dejected, her eyes glazed in helplessness. Stamped on the image of her body are the words "darkness of the heart" (*kokoro no yami*), upon which an electric bulb in the upper right corner, held by a strong, masculine hand, shines energizing light. From the rays emanate the words "Chūjōtō," suggesting that the drug was a contemporary antidote for the suffering of women. "Although the darkness of the night can be lit by lamplight," the caption reads, "the darkness of the heart of a woman suffering from illness can be lit only by Chūjōtō." The ad encourages women who are "roaming about in darkness" quickly to ease their distress by taking Chūjōtō, with which "your body will soon become strong" and "yesterday's sadness" will be transformed into "today's happiness." The ad's power emanates from its dramatization of the stark opposition between suffering and happiness, darkness and light, woman and man.

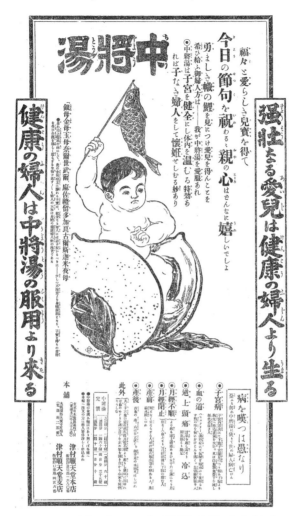

FIGURE 3.2 Advertisement for Chūjōtō, *Yomiuri shimbun*, May 5, 1909. Reproduced by permission of Tsumura & Co. and The Yomiuri Shimbun.

Advertisements for products like Chūjōtō reinforced the official gender ideology about the responsibility of women to bear and raise healthy children for the sake of the nation, but also cast light on the suffering of women pressed to fulfill such social obligations. In other words, the ads drew on what were real challenges for some women in their everyday lives. They dramatized and tapped into women's feelings of isolation, as a full-page newspaper advertisement in 1911 exemplified.[24] The ad divides the lives of women into four distinct phases: "worries of a maiden," "tears of a bride," "grief of a housewife,"

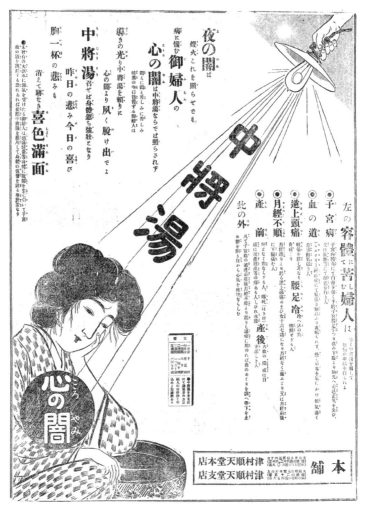

FIGURE 3.3 Full-page advertisement for Chūjōtō, *Yomiuri shimbun*, August 29, 1910. Reproduced by permission of Tsumura & Co. and The Yomiuri Shimbun.

and "pleasures of an old woman." As a maiden, a woman suffers because her illnesses scare away potential spouses. As a newlywed bride she sheds tears because

the happy dream of newlywed life fades, as [your] mother-in-law's heart chills and the pampering and treatment as a guest lasts no more than one, two, or three months after the wedding. All kinds of unkind words are spoken behind the daughter-in-law's back, and on top of that, the wife of Murata hides the illness of her lower parts out of habit, though she feels the pain inside.

The source of the pain, as described in the ad, could be found in a range of ailments, including hysteria, or "what has since the olden days been called the path of blood." The woman's mother-in-law mistakes illness for laziness, directing streams of abuse at her so that all the new bride can do is "secretly wring her kimono sleeves of her sad tears." Nor does life seem to improve as a housewife, especially if a woman cannot bear children. "At night when it is already midnight," the ad reads, "there is no sign of a husband's return and a wife, alone, is unable to contain her loneliness," made worse by an illness that prevents her from bearing children. She remains estranged from her husband who has turned to "taking his leisure at tea houses" instead of spending time in her company at home. In the final stage of womanhood, an elderly woman ought to feel pleasure, the caption reads, yet the drawing of the woman in the final frame is not a happy one—she, too, sits alone and dejected "because her body is weak [and] she remains trapped inside her home, nagging her daughter-in-law about the most insignificant things, spending one miserable day after another." The advertisement suggested that Chūjōtō will be "a woman's companion throughout her entire life," when her family failed her. Dramatizing social and familial isolation, the advertisement offered female consumers afflicted by illness and domestic distress comfort in Chūjōtō.

To be sure, the representations of women and their families in the patent medicine advertisements bordered on caricature. The advertisements drew on such widespread tropes as the "good-for-nothing-husband" who spent money recklessly, returned home in a drunken stupor, and cheated on his wife. Remarks about unforgiving mothers-in-law were common, too. Still, the ads provided visual emblems of suffering that invoked women's actual experiences within their families, especially ones that were often taken for granted. For instance, household strife, whether between wives and husbands or women and their mothers-in-law in urban and rural families alike, was a popular topic of discussion in women's magazines and newspapers. Conflicts between women and their mothers-in-law could be intense, especially for those co-residing in rural areas. Divorce rates were thus higher in the countryside. In the 1920s, there was even a correlation between living with one's in-laws and divorce rates. One of the most common reasons for divorce was articulated as a woman not being able to fit into the "ways of the house," usually a euphemism for a newlywed woman's inability to adapt to the mother-in-law's (or in some cases the husband's) expectations regarding household duties and obligations.[25]

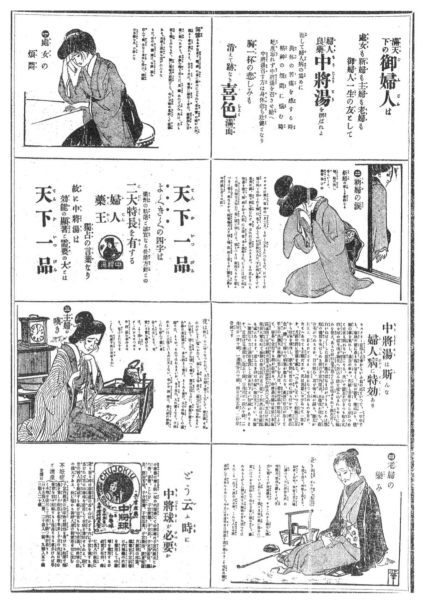

FIGURE 3.4 Full-page advertisement for Chūjōtō, *Yomiuri shimbun*, October 26, 1911. Reproduced by permission of Tsumura & Co. and The Yomiuri Shimbun.

Although the advertisements dramatized the domestic and inner lives of women, they also reflected new social and familial configurations caused by the growth of urbanization and capitalism. The population of the six largest cities—Tokyo, Yokohama, Nagoya, Osaka, Kyoto, and Kobe—had tripled from 1888 to 1918, mostly as a result of increased opportunity for industrial employment. Late nineteenth-century migrants to cities mainly worked in factories and domestic service. In the decades around World War I, white collar professionals educated in the new national schools began filling the cities, too, as large-scale businesses and the professionalization of jobs in fields such as government, education, and medicine increased the chance of basing families' livelihoods on stable, salaried employment. Distinct from the "old middle class" of small business owners, craftsmen, and traditional teachers, this "new middle class" featured men in command of the skills required by modern business, professional, and bureaucratic life and relatively educated women at the helm of domestic life. Couples no longer lived in multigenerational households among parents, relatives, and servants. Urban women did not engage in the communal tasks of harvesting, milling, or husbandry required of those living in rural areas. As suggested by the advertisements, urban middle- and upper-class women's lives centered on their relationships with their husbands, mothers-in-law, and children in a domestic space that might be seen as either liberating from the demands of intensive labor or confining in its psychological isolation.

Domesticating Hysteria in Medical Narratives

Along with producers of patent medicine advertisements, medical specialists contributed to the "domestication" of hysteria in early twentieth-century Japan by embedding it in narratives about the dangers of changes in gender and family norms. Newly minted physicians and psychiatrists began benefiting from a growing marketplace by publishing popular medical manuals, books, and pamphlets, as well as writing for magazines and newspapers, on the topic of women's health. Building on a tradition of general medical publications on dietary regimens and health originating in the Edo period, the sale and consumption of medical manuals expanded with the improved printing technologies and growing literacy rates of the late Meiji period. Hysteria was one of many new diagnoses introduced in these publications, regularly receiving entries in home encyclopedias and popular medical handbooks beginning in the late nineteenth century. Usually written by general medical practitioners or specialists, these texts targeted general audiences rather than the medical community, and in many cases were geared toward a female readership seeking instruction in managing a healthy and hygienic family and home.

Hysteria served as a convenient and expressive means of essentializing women at a time when the definition and boundaries of women's roles in society and family were being debated by a range of people. In the popular medical manuals of male physicians, hysteria could be boiled down to the essential "nature" of all women. Medical manuals like Tamura Kasaburō's *Hygiene of the Nerves* (*Shinkei no eisei*), first serialized in the *Yomiuri* newspaper in 1906 and published as a book in 1907 with multiple reprints to follow, exemplified the connection increasingly made between hysteria and the "temperament of women":

> The illness known as hysteria is usually contracted by women. Cases of male hysteria are extremely rare. For that reason, when talking about hysteria, we must be sure to talk first about the temperament of women (*fujin no seishitsu*). And since it is rather difficult to understand the nature of women, it is that much harder to understand the true nature of the illness known as hysteria. It is a strange illness—and if you cannot understand women, you cannot possibly understand hysteria.[26]

For Tamura, an understanding of hysteria required an understanding of the seemingly uniform category of women—their temperament and essence. He elaborated his essentialist conception by explaining that hysteria marked a change in a woman's natural temperament. Once happy, she became sad. Her propensity to envy intensified, her obedience and elegance diminished, and she gained in strength and roughness. "She forgets her sense of shame," Tamura wrote, "and takes a kind of pride in the bad conditions of her uterus and pays attention only to her sickness, becoming impatient and irritated with both her husband and children." Her household then fell apart because of her neglect, leading Tamura to the conclusion that "if a housewife becomes sick with this illness, a tragic illness of darkness will befall the household."[27] Most popular health manuals described hysteria along the lines of Tamura's descriptions of women's temperament, representing hysteria as a set of negative personality traits.

Another important example can be found in psychiatrist Sugie Tadasu's *Research on Hysteria and Its Treatment* (*Hisuterii no kenkyū to sono ryōhō*) (1915), a book aimed at correcting popular misperceptions of the illness. In the introduction Sugie bemoaned that the word "hysteria" was overused, with various illnesses often misdiagnosed as hysteria, and the diagnosis misused as exclusive to women. "From a medical perspective," he wrote, "there are specific, determined symptoms of hysteria" and "it is not an illness that affects only women but men and children as well."[28] His book consisted of hundreds of pages of exhaustive explanations of the causes, symptoms, prevention, and treatment of hysteria, an encyclopedic summary of the most up-to-date theories from around the world, including Freud's psychoanalytic theories about the traumatic origins of hysteria in women's experiences of childhood sexual abuse.[29] Although Sugie argued in the opening pages against the purported link between women and hysteria, the bulk of his book betrayed the same propensity to assume that the hysterical patient was most often female. He emphasized the "hysterical personality," which he explained as arguably the dimension of hysteria that affected people the most in their everyday lives and posed problems in social interactions.[30] He chose to foreground the social effects of hysteria—its impact on the family, marital, and social life—throughout the book.

The focus on women's temperament and personality among writers of medical manuals partly derived from a growing trend in German medicine to treat hysteria not as a set of physical symptoms but as a personality type. Japanese psychiatrists like Sugie tended to adopt the theories of European psychiatrists who conceived hysteria as a set of reactions of a certain type of personality. The standard psychiatry textbook after Kure's, written by Shimoda Mitsuzō and Sugita Naoki in the 1920s, stated that hysteria was a type of reaction rather than a disease: hysterical symptoms appeared when a congenitally degenerate psychopathic personality experienced psychological causes. Shimoda and Sugita wrote:

> Recently, following the opinion of many psychiatrists, hysteria is not seen as a distinct type of disease but as a kind of psychotic personality (*seishinbyōteki seikaku*) rooted in inborn abnormalities. It is said that this personality serves as the foundation to which psychological factors are added to produce the so-called symptoms of hysteria. As a result, some scholars have discarded the disease name of *hisuterii* [...] while others have stopped interpreting the word hysteria as a disease entity and understand it as simply denoting a group of hysterical symptoms.[31]

Hysteria was thus transformed from a disease into behaviors and feelings that characterized the self's relationship with and reaction to others in the world, as well as to oneself.[32] Psychiatrists began to speak less about the intensity of the stress of hysterical fits and more about the underlying personality.

The adoption of the personality-focused theory of hysteria must be understood in the context of broader changes related to women and gender identity in the early twentieth century. The expansion of women's education and employment, exposure to new models of marriage and family life, and the growth of a middle class fueled popular debate on the "women's problem" (*fujin mondai*) in the early decades of the twentieth century. The debate centered on the figure of the "new woman" that emerged from early feminist writings in the early 1910s. The "new woman" exuded what feminist social critic Itō Noe called in 1913 "a firm self-confidence" and an emotional independence from the patriarchal family.[33] Although the debate, which focused on the dignity of separate spheres and the nature of maternal love, had little effect on familiar ideology, it drew attention to an assertive femininity that led part of the reading public to reconsider the Meiji legacy of sexual hierarchy and discrimination.[34]

For some, talk of feminine self-assertion sparked fears of grave social consequences. Doctors like Sugie and Tamura were among the critics who spoke despairingly of the continually blurring distinctions between males and females as well as the prescribed norm of devotion to family for women. One of the "emotional impairments" that ensued in a case of hysteria, Sugie argued, was the way women flouted social obligations for the sake of unsanctioned and passionate love:

> You often see a hysterical person abandoning her parents, abandoning her home, and in the worst cases forgetting her duties and reputation to lose her way in the darkness of love. In the end she is seized by a momentary curiosity, misled by vanity, and weakened emotionally by absurd thoughts. She becomes a thing of love. Her life becomes awash in an unrecoverable dishonor. Among people who stain a family's name or make a husband lose face, many are individuals with hysteria, or ladies with status and education who face unexpected scandal and who are crushed in society by their immorality. These kinds of people, when it comes to love, are potentially a great danger.[35]

Sugie's concerns about the immorality of scandalous women were shared by contemporary social reformers worried about the increase in domestic social problems in the decade after the Russo-Japanese War (1904–1905).[36] Victorious in war but wracked by violent strikes as the economy descended into a postwar recession, Japan faced an array of social problems. Ideologues of all stripes expressed concerns about the moral fiber of citizens, with socialists advocating radical political change, nihilists questioning any established moral system in the face of a hopeless world, and state officials bemoaning the decline of Japanese youth as the reason for the social ills of the time. Minister of Education Makino Nobuaki's 1906 "Fūki kunrei" (Morals Directive) was directed at students who he thought were straying from the ideals of "whole-some thoughts" and "concrete goals," and falling prey to socialism, decadence, and petty concerns. Makino blamed the moral decline for the flood of "recently published writings and images" that overstimulated the impressionable minds of young readers and propelled them toward various forms of unwholesome behavior.[37] "Makino thus established a direct link between the moral decline of students and the technological and commercial advances in the late-Meiji publishing industry, which produced a heavy stream of books, magazines, and newspapers."[38]

Sugie, too, blamed popular plays and novels for the encouragement of the "emotional impairments" that led to love scandals. Women, he wrote, went to the theaters and read novels where "this [scandalous] way of feeling" is presented in the extreme. Female viewers admired the characters and scenery, responding with tears gushing forth and becoming so drunken with various imagined fantasies that in the end "the pure body is offered as sacrifice to evil spirits."[39] Imaginations ran wild so that women could not distinguish between fiction and reality. Sugie gave an example of a girl who saw a performance of "Awa no naruto," and suddenly remembered that she, too, was separated from her parents at birth and sent forth as a child on a pilgrimage of the Shikoku temples. She then ran away from home to visit her birth parents. "These young girls," Sugie lamented, "with no experience in society are easily led astray by their imaginations" and ultimately made mistakes when choosing their husbands or waiting too long to marry.[40]

Medical handbooks thus defined hysteria not only as a disease but as an explanation for transgressive behavior that violated the norms of gender hierarchy and family expectations. Sugie interpreted such behavior not as a product of structural changes but as the pathology of individual personality. Women were becoming increasingly selfish and flouting their received roles, he wrote, because of the spread of what he deemed pathological personalities. As suggested by his near-caricature descriptions of hysterical women falling victim to their imaginations and posing a danger to society, Sugie and other male physicians linked hysteria with women in a context of heightened anxieties about the viability of the so-called traditional family and conventional gender roles, as well as the perceived crisis of national decadence. Their popular books and pamphlets often turned out to be conservative social critiques disguised as medical claims to knowledge. Their medical writings for popular audiences expressed a cultural narrative about the dangers of social change and the role of gender as a politicized category for interpreting new social relationships and identities.

Multiple Sites of Treatment

Authors of popular medical manuals were not alone in taking advantage of a booming market for healing therapies. Between the mid-1910s and early 1930s, entrepreneurs, medical professionals, self-stylized healers, and government officials offered therapies that extended sites of care from the home to an eclectic array of places. Hospitals, clinics, rest homes, counseling centers, police-sponsored personal consultation offices, local organizations of mental healers, temples, hot springs, offices of the New Religions—all became available to middle- and upper-class consumers in search of remedies for various forms of sufferings of the heart and mind.[41]

The meanings and practices created by the marketplace of healing were differentiated by gender. Self-healing, for instance, was associated primarily with men. Women may have purchased patent medicines or consulted home encyclopedias and women's magazines for guidelines and advice, but they were seen as the recipients of remedies for health. By contrast, men were regarded as the creators of forms of self-healing in a commodified world popularly known as "mental healing" (*seishin ryōhō*). In this world, men both produced and consumed a mix of meditation, dietary regimens, deep breathing exercises, massage, and other techniques to awaken the powers of the mind and cure the mind and body of such ailments as neurasthenia, all without consulting a doctor or entering a hospital.[42] Hundreds of different approaches to mental healing circulated in the 1910s and 1920s, many invented by university-educated male writers, bureaucrats, scientists, doctors, and intellectuals who offered instruction in the techniques they pioneered.[43] They founded organizations in both rural and urban areas, with disciples later establishing branches as well. Some of the organizations resembled contemporary institutions of higher learning, self-identifying as a "college" or "university" and issuing certificates upon the completion of training courses. Others were modeled on the *iemoto* (literally, "the foundation of the family") system common among lineages of artists in which a male master who had inherited his position either through shared kinship or selection by the previous master instructed disciples below him.[44] "Mental healing" was a commercialized and institutionalized industry of men.

Women and men seeking cures for mental distress turned to healers among the so-called New Religions, too. Distinct from the "established religions" of temple Buddhism, shrine Shinto, and Christianity, New Religions had begun appearing since the middle of the nineteenth century, with another cluster emerging in the 1920s and 1930s. They usually originated with the revelations of a highly charismatic founder, many of them women, who attracted their followers through healing and other "this-worldly benefits," including solutions to family problems and material prosperity. Although many new religions had their original bases in rural areas, they rapidly expanded into towns and cities throughout the country. As the example of a popular sect called Hitonomichi Kyōdan suggests, the popular appeal of many New Religions derived from their incorporation of many aspects of urban modernity into their activities and teachings. Historians Yamano Haruo and Narita Ryūichi have shown how Hitonomichi Kyōdan encouraged husbands and wives to spend more time together in a context of a shift from three-generation households to nuclear families in cities. The organization sponsored "couples' discussion groups" and its clerics emphasized the importance of sexual love as the key to a happy marriage, attracting followers among many women (and men) into the 1930s.[45]

The explosion of healing therapies in the early decades of the twentieth century is usually explained as a sign of disillusionment with Western-derived biomedical science, which emphasized the biological aspects of health and disease, and a resulting turn toward "alternative" approaches that emphasized nonmaterial and transcendent factors—the human spirit (*seishin*), cosmic energy, divinity—in sustaining health. Similar to contemporary Europeans and Americans who began turning to the occult sciences, mind cure, and Spiritualism, many Japanese sought succor from "alternative" therapies. They deftly combined imported practices like hypnotism with indigenous techniques of bodily and spiritual discipline, including meditative techniques to awaken the powers of mind and body, to produce what was popularly called "mental healing" (*seishin ryōhō*). Historians have suggested that the mental healing movement in Japan emerged as a form of "alternative knowledge" at a time when science was reaching the peak of its hegemony, reordering everyday life to the detriment of "folk" and "religious" knowledge.[46] It is true that even physicians expressed concerns about the limitations of biomedicine, namely its neglect of the person as a being made up by far more than their biological functions. In the 1910s and beyond, doubts about the efficacy and authority of officially sanctioned institutions of medical science wafted in the air.

Yet ordinary consumers did not necessarily rely on a distinction between "orthodox" and "alternative" therapies when seeking treatment for mental and spiritual illnesses. Nor did they always regard such state-supported institutions of medical care as the hospital as the most desirable sites of care. Regardless of official hierarchies created by state officials and medical professions, factors such as cost and location influenced consumer choice more significantly in the marketplace of healing. The primary clientele of hospitals, for instance, consisted of affluent members of the upper and middle classes, especially with the proliferation of private hospitals in urban areas that competed intensely with one another for patients and profit. Hospital care proved too expensive for most Japanese, with a month-long stay in one private hospital costing more than half the monthly salary of an urban, white collar company employee or government bureaucrat.[47] Members of the lower classes were limited to either qualifying for prefectural government–subsidized care in public and private hospitals or resorting to quarantine hospitals established for sufferers of infectious diseases like tuberculosis, syphilis, cholera, and leprosy.

The decision to seek medical care at hospitals was influenced by cultural and gendered understandings of this relatively new site of care. Although many hospitals had evolved from the abandoned temple buildings housing ten or fewer patients of the 1870s to the multistory brick properties with wards for hundreds of patients of the 1920s, the reasons for avoiding hospital-based treatment persisted. In the popular imagination, hospitals remained, on the one hand, privileged sites of care for the affluent, but on the other hand, institutions of exploitation. In 1904, Meiji physician Kondō Tsunejirō criticized the commercial and restrictive nature of hospitals by comparing them to brothels and prisons:

> As for the [private] hospital, it is exactly like a brothel that is greedy for profit. . . . As for the public hospital, it is nothing more than another form of the prison. The attitudes of the hospital director and the revered and distinguished doctors beneath him are indeed intimidating. They view the sick person as a criminal. When the doctors make their rounds, they question the patient about his symptoms, just like a public prosecutor interrogating a suspect.[48]

Searing critique aside, Kondo was not alone in his concern about the transformation of treatment into commodity, patient into customer or criminal in the context of the early twentieth-century hospital. A series of exposés in the *Yomiuri* newspaper in 1901 uncovered the abuse and corruption occurring in seven psychiatric hospitals across Tokyo, censuring the collusions of medicine and business. One historian of medicine has concluded that modern medicine in Meiji Japan was "nothing other than a process of subordinating medicine to capitalism," shaped by the shifting political arrangements between private doctors and the state.[49]

Misgivings about hospital-based care help explain the appeal of self-diagnosis and self-treatment, especially among women, and the vulnerability of sufferers to the many advertisers of patent medicines and authors of home medical manuals. One article-length infomercial for Chūjōtō described the possible attitudes and circumstances of three groups of women who would benefit from home treatment. The first group consisted of women who were unaware of their own illnesses and believed that "[all] women simply have vaginal discharge (*koshige*), naturally get cold, and have headaches in accordance with the seasons." The author continued, "women who are not blessed with children think that there is no path left for them, and even when something is wrong with their body they do not realize it and put off receiving treatment." The second group included women who feared treatment: "you know you are sick and that something is wrong with your body. You want to receive treatment but fear that your mother-in-law will criticize you for being weak and so you refrain from complaining, delay treatment, and ultimately feel worse." There were also women who desired treatment, but felt embarrassed about visiting a doctor who will "examine all sorts of places on your body." The final group consisted of women who could not receive treatment for the practical reason that they were too busy or too few doctors practiced in their neighborhoods, especially in rural areas.[50] "The solution," the ad claimed, "is home treatment! There is nothing difficult about home treatment. [Chūjōtō] is a perfect drinkable medicine that has been tested by many famous gynecologists and has produced good results." The ad emphasized that self-treatment at home provided women the privacy and discretion unavailable in hospitals and clinics.

Meanwhile, recent young male graduates of the nation's many medical schools as well as private entrepreneurs and social reformers began opening private clinics and hospitals, often replacing the prefectural and municipal hospitals that closed due to lack of funding. The Kyoto Prefectural Asylum, for instance, closed its doors a mere seven years after its establishment in 1875 by a local civic activist and a doctor. Local businesses and village elites soon joined forces to establish the Private Iwakura Asylum, renamed the Iwakura Psychiatric Hospital in 1892.[51] Competition for patients was fierce among various hospitals in urban areas, with advertisements for hospitals "promising such things as 'the complete cure of epilepsy in seventeen days'" becoming a standard fixture in newspapers and magazines.[52] The growth of medical specialties related to women's health contributed to the growth of clinics and hospitals catering toward women. They advertised their knowledge and services not only through print advertisements, but also by answering questions submitted by housewives and other female readers to the "Hygiene Consultation" columns in national newspapers. For families seeking mental-health care who were either affluent enough to pay the hospital fees or poor enough to qualify for public assistance, private psychiatric hospitals, clinics, and centers became increasingly common sites of care.

Women's Narratives of "Hysteria" in a Family Vernacular

In early twentieth-century Japanese psychiatric hospitals and other similar sites of care, methods of close observation and documentation created opportunities for psychiatrists, nurses, and patients to narrate experiences of sickness.[53] Patient files contained logbooks in which doctors and nurses transcribed selections of interviews with patients about their sickness, family life, reasons for hospitalization, and more.[54] Fragments of their often-cryptic conversations littered the pages. "Why did you throw the nurse out [of your room] yesterday," asked the Medical Director of a thirty-two-year-old woman, to which she responded, "I am not that troublesome. Why send a nurse?" On another day, in response to the examining psychiatrist Suzuki's question of "How about the time that you entered the hospital?" she said, "I thought I was being admitted even though I was not sick, but now that some time has passed, I think I cannot leave [this place]. I think I was, indeed, sick." Suzuki further inquired, "Sick in what way?" and she is said to have responded by indicating the reckless way in which she would become upset and the way she would throw and break items.[55] The doctors and nurses, of course, selectively recorded parts of conversations, making it difficult to ascertain the content of omissions, but the dialogue nonetheless reveal patterns among patients' responses (the frequent use of the word "sick," for instance, rather than "mentally ill") and idiomatic turns of phrase.

The materials in patient files contributed to the growth of an oral and written culture of self-expression among the afflicted that circulated beyond the walls of the hospital. Psychiatrists published analyses of the handwriting of patients in medical journals. Drawings and poetry by patients appeared in standard psychiatry textbooks.[56] Once discharged, former patients published memoirs and autobiographies.[57] Journalists interviewed patients about their experience in the hospital.[58] The words and images of the afflicted certainly had exotic appeal, but the first-person accounts also gained ground in a broader cultural and literary context that elevated the direct expression of lived experience. From the so-called I-novel that mobilized "the special mystique of the notion of *watakushi*" to the popular genre of confessional writing, modes of expression that featured self-exploration and autobiography, whether in fiction or nonfiction, were increasingly extolled as more truthful and more "Japanese" in comparison to "fictional" and "imaginative" Western novels.[59]

One significant archive of writings by women and men overcoming nervous illness originated in a new and uncommon site of psychiatric care of the 1920s and 1930s known as the "therapy home" or "rest home" (*ryōhōjyo*). Therapy homes offered psychotherapy, a relatively unpopular approach to treating psychological distress in Japanese psychiatry where biological understandings of mental disease dominated. One of the first psychiatrists to produce theories about the psychological origins—as opposed to biological or organic causes—of nervous illness was Morita Masatake, a student of Kure Shūzō's. Based on his experiences working with Kure at Sugamo Hospital and in treating his own nervous condition as well as those of friends inside his home, Morita concluded that this type of suffering arose from a natural disposition toward neurosis (*shinkeishitsu*), curable only by relinquishing attempts at regulating the mind with thoughts and intentions and instead learning to live in relationship with reality "as it is" (*aru ga mama*). Morita operated a therapy clinic inside Negishi Hospital in Tokyo, the private psychiatric hospital where he had become the medical director in 1906.

Around the same time, literary critic–turned-doctor Nakamura Kokyō also began providing in-patient psychotherapy, first without a medical license in the Shinagawa neighborhood of Tokyo in the late 1910s and then in a rest home in the suburb of Chiba after 1929. Nakamura's rest home, later called the Nakamura Kokyō Ryōhōjo and now Nakamura Kokyō Memorial Hospital, consisted of four residences with gardens and a small barn in the 1930s. Between 1929 and 1932, Nakamura possibly treated over 200 patients, a range of men and women who seem to have belonged mostly to the middle and upper classes from both rural and urban areas. Male university students, wives of government bureaucrats and company employees, men running family businesses, and vocational school students found their way to Nakamura's rest home after having tried various other methods of healing and usually at the urging of a family member or friend.[60]

A balance of activity and introspection, all to be documented in writing, lay at the heart of Nakamura and Morita's psychotherapeutic approaches.[61] Both treatments involved four stages—seclusion and rest, light occupational therapy, heavy occupational therapy, and complex activities—interspersed with lectures, reading, and writing. Patients were required to write diary entries about the day's activities and changes in their thoughts and feelings, which were submitted to the psychiatrists for commentary. Patient diaries were published in specialist medical journals, serving as data and case studies for doctors and others studying and healing nervous illnesses. Morita regularly published diary entries in his medical journal *Shinkeishitsu*, with more than forty diaries appearing between 1930 and 1940 as well as about fifty letters of consultation written by patients and Morita's responses to them. Unlike Morita, Nakamura showcased excerpts of patient diaries in his newspaper articles, magazine features, and books aimed at non-specialist, popular audiences. Through a series of articles on hysteria in 1928 and 1929 in the most widely read women's magazine *Shufu no tomo* (Housewife's Friend), and a book published in 1932 by the magazine's publishing house based on the series, Nakamura became the period's best-known medical expert on hysteria.[62]

For readers of *Shufu no tomo*, Nakamura presented his therapeutic method as a gentle, non-invasive, and effective way of overcoming illness. Consider a visual narrative of photographs and excerpts from one woman's daily diary published by *Shufu no tomo*. The narrative moves readers frame by frame through the various stages of the woman's treatment in his rest home. In the opening frames, the woman lies on her *futon*, or mattress, with a blanket covering her face. She looks down as she strokes her hair in front of a mirror. Quotes from her diary entry included as captions to the images reveal that she is unhappy and desolate in this moment. In the following frames, she leaves behind the isolation of the bedroom into the open yard underneath wide skies where she feeds chicks, scrubs floors, and weeds a garden. Lest the reader think the woman might be feeling better, though, the captions, again culled from her daily dairy, indicate that she feels uneasy, either because of her sickness (*byōki*) or her concerns for her children. The work is not easy. "If I were at home," she writes, "my servants would do all the chores, but here in the rest home, you have to work, whether you feel good or bad." Soon enough, the woman begins to enjoy her tasks, writing that she is "grateful [that] a body as weak as mine has come to be able to work (*kunren*) like this every day."[63] Her stay at the rest home has removed the woman from her usual domestic context filled with servants and children, which has supposedly deprived her of the joys of working with her own hands.

The overseer of the work in the romanticized rural backdrop of the rest home was none other than the male *sensei*, or doctor-teacher. As the woman in the visual narrative is slowly socialized into the rhythms and tasks of communal life, she and others tend to plants as Nakamura stands behind

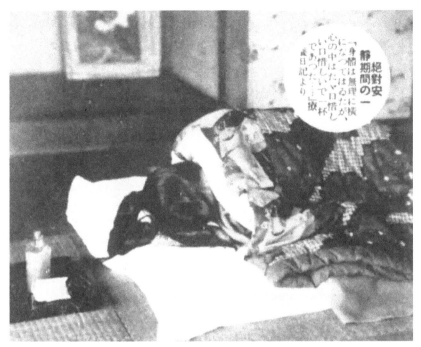

FIGURE 3.5 Visual narrative of an anonymous woman's treatment in a rest home in the late 1920s. Reproduced from Nakamura Kokyō, *Hisuterii no ryōhō* (Tokyo: Shufu no tomo sha, 1932).

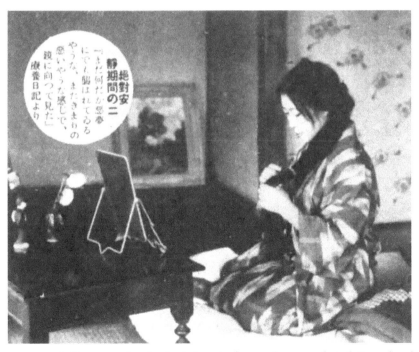

FIGURE 3.6 The woman brushes her hair and reflects on her state of mind. Reproduced from Nakamura Kokyō, *Hisuterii no ryōhō* (Tokyo: Shufu no tomo sha, 1932).

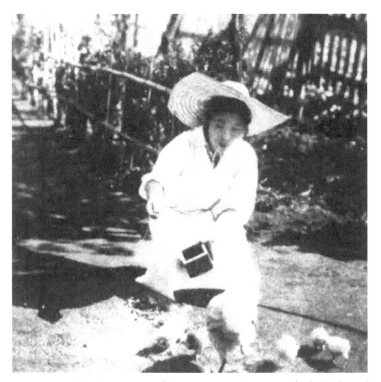

FIGURE 3.7 As the next part of her treatment, the woman feeds chicks and performs other outdoor chores by herself. Reproduced from Nakamura Kokyō, *Hisuterii no ryōhō* (Tokyo: Shufu no tomo sha, 1932).

the female patients with their identical hats working in the garden or fields. He is charged with guiding the women in their *kunren*, or disciplinary practice of the mind and body, a notion derived from religious and spiritual traditions of mind cultivation.[64] As a result of her *kunren*, the woman featured in the narrative is depicted as having achieved by the end of her stay a form of self-knowledge that enables her to compose herself, both in writing and in mind, in the final frame. No longer disheveled in appearance and anxious in mind, she writes that she has come to realize that her "illness" had been caused by her feelings and approach to life. By removing herself from the space of her biological family and taking refuge in that of a temporary chosen family of fellow patients led by the patriarchal figure of the male doctor, the woman is depicted as having exhibited the industriousness in manual and emotional labor necessary to attain self-awareness and self-inscription through writing.

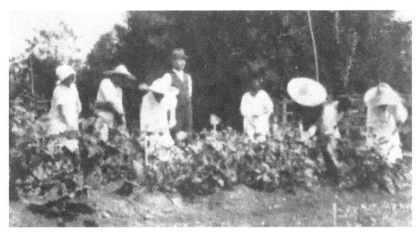

FIGURE 3.8 The woman moves on to participate in communal work, with Dr. Nakamura Kokyō overseeing the women's progress. Reproduced from Nakamura Kokyō, *Hisuterii no ryōhō* (Tokyo: Shufu no tomo sha, 1932).

It is possible that some women in Nakamura's rest home achieved such a form of self-knowledge, but some accounts suggest that female patients and doctors offered parallel, or even incommensurable, narratives about the causes and effects of the women's mental and emotional ailments. In late 1929, a thirty-four-year-old woman in the rest home revealed her side of the story to Nakamura in the form of a confessional letter that exposed the complexities of kinship and family in which her sufferings were embedded. Her husband, a white collar company employee, and her mother had accompanied her to Nakamura's rest home, insisting that she stay to find a cure for her nervous breakdowns, during which she babbled nonsense, became highly excitable, and felt deep jealousy. Her husband and mother had informed Nakamura that the woman had already received various treatments. A gynecologist had diagnosed her with a uterine infection (endometritis), but the treatment did not cure her babbling. Meeting with a famous mountain ascetic (*yamashi bōzu*) seemed to help at first, but the symptoms returned later in the year. In the words of her husband, his wife's convulsive attacks had been provoked by "a family matter" in which she had learned of his former engagement to another woman. The woman's mother interrupted her son-in-law here to declare: "All of this is entirely my fault. I raised her as a spoiled child. I feel truly sorry for him [points to her son-in-law]. Since the spring, he has worried in ways that are indescribable about my daughter's illness. Even his face and body have visibly thinned."[65] Through this public performance, the mother of

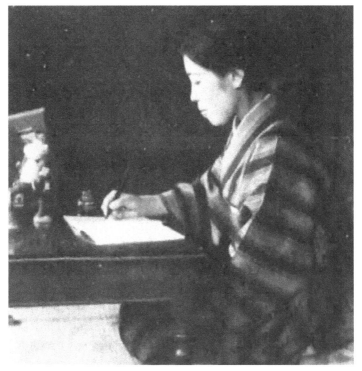

FIGURE 3.9 The fully recovered woman writes in her diary the evening before she leaves the rest home. Reproduced from Nakamura Kokyō, *Hisuterii no ryōhō* (Tokyo: Shufu no tomo sha, 1932).

the afflicted woman deploys a common cultural and social script that elevates the actions of the husband/son-in-law at the expense of her own daughter's. The daughter, Nakamura writes, spoke not a single word but glared at both her husband and mother throughout the conversation.

She was not silent for long. After four weeks of treatment in the rest home, she wrote and submitted to Nakamura a long letter instead of her daily diary entry in which she asked for his guidance: "You may laugh at how trifling the incident was," she writes in an intimate and even confessional tone, "but to you only, *sensei*, I will reveal everything in my heart. I cannot but tell you all of this frankly."[66] She described her "illness" as a decade—not a few months, as her mother and husband had declared—in the making, beginning with her husband's temporary relocation to Taiwan for work, when he had had an affair with the head nurse of the Red Cross in Taiwan, a woman who happened to be his first cousin. The patient and her husband had long been mired in a thick web of familial and social obligations with this cousin. Her husband financially supported his cousin's family, lending money to her brothers to support their education and business ventures. Upon learning about the affair, the woman admitted to Nakamura's rest home felt angry and frustrated, especially when the cousin asked again for more financial support. But she wrote that she suffered alone, not daring to reveal her suspicions to her husband, though she did consult her mother and mother-in-law.

Although Nakamura diagnosed the woman with hysteria, she was either unaware of the diagnosis or implicitly rejected it as a way in which to understand her state of mind and body. When she experienced her first convulsive attack, she had long been aware of her husband's indiscretions and had recently learned about his former fiancée as well:

> Everything in front of my eyes went black, my chest throbbed as if it were about to burst, my body started to shake, and my mouth would not work. Without even a moment to think about what was happening, I was already in so much pain that I could not remain standing. I fell over on my side and no sooner had that happened, my whole body stiffened as hard as a rod. My husband and children bent over me and pressed down on me, but to no avail. (This is grand seizure hysteria).[67]

The parenthetical remark was added by Nakamura, who interpreted the woman's symptoms in the language of medical etiology. The woman, on the other hand, revealed at this point in her letter that the initial spasms opened her mind and heart to a world of memories that she had long repressed. She recalled that her husband was, in fact, a distant cousin of hers, and that their families had known one another for decades. She had been promised to him when she was fourteen years old. She remembered that he had been highly sought after by many women and that he had become involved with another woman during their engagement, which had nearly broken off their marriage because it had sent her father into a rage. She referred to her "sickness" frequently in the letter, often describing it as both physical and psychological in origin and effects. Not once did she use the term "hysteria," but instead invoked references to her "heart" (*kokoro*) as the object of suffering: "my heart fell sick," she wrote, or "it pained my heart."[68] Women diagnosed with hysteria by their families or in psychiatric hospitals, too, often rejected the concept, arguing instead that their ailments originated in their masculine tendencies or domestic circumstances.[69] For these women, the concept of hysteria seemed neither to help them make sense of their social and personal experiences nor to help them cope with and resolve practical questions.

By contrast, Nakamura insisted on the pathological nature of his patient's spasms and babbling. He wrote in his response, "As I've mentioned from time to time during lectures and talks, [spasms and babbling] are shameful, pathological (*byōteki*), mentally abnormal phenomena." He explained that she could overcome them if she disciplined her mind more thoroughly. "Through your own willpower (*iryoku*), you can avoid [these symptoms]." He explained in a moralizing tone how "the things that go on between man and wife, or any relation, are not simply the responsibility of the two people involved but the sin (*tsumi*) of many, many people, all humans, even myself."[70] He instructed her to approach her experience of ten years "reasonably, charitably, and compromisingly."[71] To some extent, Nakamura implied that his rest home provided the space but not the cure for the woman's sufferings. Instead he drew on a broader cultural and spiritual discourses with origins in earlier centuries on forms of "discipline" (*kunren*) that could help women and men will themselves to health and happiness.[72] Nakamura did not seem interested in asking his female patients to delve deeply into their past domestic, familial, and sexual experiences, as one might presume of early twentieth-century psychotherapists. Yet the same women insisted on making sense of the personal and family circumstances in which they had reached the brink of psychic breakdown. At times they deployed an intimate family vernacular in their interactions with the doctor, too, addressing him as an authoritative male confidant, as if he were simultaneously a professional figure and friend, a patriarch and intimate partner. The family vernacular in which women spoke and wrote thus compels a reading of the archive of hysteria that recognizes but also disassembles the medical and psychotherapeutic framework, one that tended to pathologize rather than socially contextualize women's suffering.

Although urban, middle- and upper-class women took advantage of such new sites of treatment outside the home as "rest homes" and psychiatric hospitals in the early twentieth century, they did not necessarily leave behind the intimate cultures and structures of domestic life that shaped their mental and emotional afflictions. In a family vernacular, the women described to a range of healers the thick web of domestic and social obligations in which they were embedded. Female patients interacted with examining physicians, psychotherapists, and religious specialists in ways that evoked conventional gendered intimacies and hierarchies of family. Male doctors assumed the role of an all-knowing male head-of-household who did not necessarily replace the female patient's father, husband, or brother, but instead served as extensions of family-based patriarchal care.

Women, especially those from rural areas and with less expendable income, could not always step outside the home to seek treatment. Instead, they took advantage of mail-order patent medicine and other forms of self-treatment. These women certainly were aware of the discourse of hysteria, for many heard the term deployed by their mothers, husbands, and fathers, as well as in popular discourse. But many implicitly refused to naturalize the term, the family vernacular suggesting that no single term could contain the myriad intimacies and complexities of their experiences. In their narratives, it is possible to see how popular ascription of hysteria to such factors as individual temperament and sex belied its social and familial roots.

Yet family-based care, as well as the gendered family vernacular in which women described their experiences of illness, did have their limits. Some women (and men) suffered from mental afflictions so severe that they could not be managed through a combination of home- and hospital-based care. If their behavior was socially disruptive enough, as in cases of violent crime, the family was compelled to relinquish their caretaking and custodial role to local government officials.

4
_____

Periodic Crimes in the Courtroom

ON THE EVENING of April 15 sometime during the Taisho era (1912–1926), a twenty-seven-year-old woman living near Kyoto sat in her room, thinking about the quarrel with her mother earlier that day. The quarrel had, in her words, "put her in a bad mood" (*kibun wo waruku shimashita*). Besieged with thought, sleep eluded her. She would later explain to a forensic psychiatrist, "I thought about my age, people who were younger than me who had already married, how I had not been able to marry, how I made my parents worry." Tears flowed and pain wracked her head as she headed out of her room and toward the light emanating from an electric bulb inside the room in which her mother and father slept. Then the unthinkable, both for her and others who would later assess her actions, happened: "my head started to hurt. I felt shivers. I then flared up (*gyakujō*, literally "up into reverse"), felt extremely irritated (*kan ga tatte*, literally "my nerves stood up"), and there was nothing I could do about it. I went out into the garden and grabbed a piece of wood." Before she realized what she was doing, she had struck several fatal blows with the wooden pole to her mother's head and injured her father.[1] In the months that followed, she and members of her family were questioned by judges, prosecutors, and expert witnesses during a prolonged trial in the Kyoto District Court. There was no question that she had committed murder, but this was not enough to hold her legally responsible for the crime. The determining factor would be her state of mind at the time of the crime—or, more precisely in the case of many female defendants, the state of her body.

Beginning in the 1910s, Japanese criminologists and jurists began contributing to legal and medical discourses about the effects of women's physiologies on their mental capacity that were circulating around the world.[2] For reasons both distinct from and similar to their counterparts in, for example, Brazil or England, Japanese forensic psychiatrists, criminologists,

Madness in the Family. H. Yumi Kim, Oxford University Press. © Oxford University Press 2022.
DOI: 10.1093/oso/9780197507353.003.0005

lawyers, and jurists more or less agreed that women's reproductive functions, especially menstruation and pregnancy, diminished their capacity for reason, propelling them toward uncontrollable crimes of passion.[3] So when a woman was put on trial for committing a crime, whether murder or petty theft, she was often asked by judges, lawyers, and expert witnesses to describe her menstrual cycle. Had she been ovulating at the time of the crime? Could she describe how she usually felt while menstruating? They promoted the theory that menstruating women were susceptible to mental disorders and psychological instability that made them prone to crime. Defense lawyers sometimes used this reasoning as a strategy to relieve women of all or partial responsibility. They did so by invoking Article 39 of the new Criminal Code of 1907, which spelled out an insanity defense that prevented the punishment of individuals who, by reason of mental "incompetency," could not fairly be held responsible for their crimes. The court hired forensic psychiatrists as expert witnesses to conduct psychiatric assessments of the women in order to determine whether the terms of Article 39 applied. If a psychiatrist diagnosed the defendant with mental "incompetency" triggered by menstruation, she might receive a reduced sentence, or even no punishment at all.

Cases of violent crime committed by women exposed the limits of the Japanese state's reliance on families as the primary caretakers and custodians of those considered mad in the early twentieth century. Some violence proved too disruptive and lethal to be contained within and by families, especially those in urban areas where cramped living quarters could not accommodate confinement rooms and neighborhood residents were less tightly bound by a sense of collective obligation toward one another. Family also could not function as the liable unit in cases of crime in the context of the creation of a new criminal code from the 1870s to 1907, which delineated notions of responsibility and culpability that differed from those in the custom-based legal system of the preceding Edo period. Families and even inter-household groups within villages had once been held collectively responsible for the crimes committed by a mentally disturbed member.[4] The newly codified Criminal Code of 1907 designated individuals—not families—as bearers of responsibility for crime. Violent crime thus exposed the limits of the state's reliance on families in the management of those considered mad.

The individuation of crime involved differentiating between the gendered bodies of women and men. The menstrual mood-disorder defense justified on medical and legal grounds the idea that women's bodily processes diminished their capacity for reason and propelled them toward uncontrollable acts of passion.[5] Such theories about the bodily processes of women causing mental and psychological abnormalities had long circulated in Japan and elsewhere, but they gained particular traction in the early twentieth century with the global rise of the sciences of sexology and criminology in the 1920s and 1930s.[6] When asked to serve as witnesses to the crime or the character of the defendant, families, too, drew on the notion that women could not fully control their bodies and behaviors due to their reproductive system.[7] Specialists and families alike rarely, if ever, portrayed men's reproductive systems as exerting as much influence over their bodies. As with hysteria, the invocation of menstrual mood disorders reduced women's psychic lives and behaviors to explanations of reproductive function. The diagnosis suggested that women's psychic and emotional lives were inseparable from the functions of their bodies.

Yet the madness allegedly induced by a woman's body proved unstable and ambiguous in the space of the criminal courtroom. Legal scholars, jurists, lawyers, and psychiatrists argued over definitions and terminologies for madness in the process of codifying the nation's criminal law in ways that cemented but also strained the emerging relationship between psychiatry and law.[8] Female defendants, too, offered understandings of their bodies that resonated with but also complicated expert testimonies and popular discourse. In forensic psychiatric reports submitted to the Kyoto District Courts in the 1920s, excerpts of interviews of female defendants reveal the complex family dynamics, gender relations, and sexual violence informing the criminal acts of the women, as well as the women's awareness of the menstrual psychosis defense and its juridical and social uses. The set of shared assumptions and language concerning menstruation suggests that the women were, in part, adapting an ever-evolving cultural script about women and their bodily functions by using a much older language of "bloody inversion," or the experience of upheavals of nervous energies and blood flows in women's bodies. As the young woman who attacked her parents described, she "flared up" and her nerves "stood up" in the moment before she committed murder. Women often invoked the language of "bloody inversion" to suggest that their bodies and behaviors were intimately connected to those within their family and kin networks. In the context of a judicial process that aimed to individuate a female defendant's body as much as possible, the women themselves used the language of "bloody inversion" in ways that bolstered notions of individual autonomy found in psychiatric and legal discourse and yet also offered distinct understandings of their allegedly mad criminal acts as having emanated from embodied experiences within the domain of kinship.

Contests between Law and Psychiatry

The adjudication of women's bodies and behaviors in the criminal courts of the 1920s and 1930s occurred in the wake of a series of contests among lawmakers and psychiatrists. Beginning in the 1890s, reforms in criminal law gave psychiatrists a limited but definite place in an evolving legal system. From the 1880s to 1900s, Meiji government officials and legal scholars strove to establish a legal system that conformed to international standards and assured foreign powers of the reliability of Japan's courts and legal codes. The government issued its first Criminal Code on July 17, 1880, which abolished key features of Edo law, including discrimination based on social status and various forms of the death penalty. Under the influence of French legal scholar Gustave Boissonade, the Code was modeled on the French Penal Code of 1810.[9] As in most European penal codes of the time, the clause on insanity in the French version left the definition of insanity open to interpretation. "There can be no crime, or delict," Article 64 of the French Penal Code began, "where the accused was in a state of madness (*démence*) at the time of the action; or when he has been constrained by a force which he had not the power to resist."[10] Similarly, the 1880 Japanese Code stated in Article 78, "There is no crime to consider if the accused was not able to distinguish between right and wrong at the time of the crime due to a loss of perception and mind (*chikaku seishin*)."[11] The origin of the legal phrase "loss of perception and mind" remains unclear; it derived neither from early psychiatric discourse nor from vernacular expressions for madness.

Legal scholars and psychiatrists quickly called for revisions to the phrase "loss of perception and mind," prompting a detailed debate about vocabularies of madness that illuminated the overlapping yet competing terms of the law and psychiatry. In 1893, psychiatrist Katayama Kunika, a professor of forensic medicine at Tokyo Imperial University, advised a commission in charge of general revisions to the Criminal Code that "perception and mind" was redundant, for "mind" already encompassed "perception."[12] Nor did madness involve a "loss" of certain faculties but rather an "abnormality" (*henjō*) that struck the mind. He suggested instead the somewhat unwieldy phrase, "a typically incurable and serious disease of the mind" (*hotondo fuchi jūdai naru seishin no shitsubyō*) as a replacement for "a loss of perception and mind."

Between 1882 and 1907, the insanity defense underwent a series of changes as the Ministry of Justice drafted five revisions of the Code, four of which were debated in the Diet. In the 1890s, the drafters consulted psychiatrists and physicians to produce the following revision in the insanity defense clause for the second version in 1894: "The act of a person who has lost his mind (*seishin wo sōshitsu shitaru mono*) is not considered a crime; a person with mental illness (*seishinbyō*) will in accordance to circumstances be subject to confinement." This was the first use of the medical term "mental illness" (*seishinbyō*) to refer to madness in a legal code.

Katayama further demanded that the law integrate medical understandings of mental disorder, which was characterized in the early twentieth century by the existence of gradations and spectra of madness. Mental disability (*seishin shōgai*) encompassed both longer-lasting forms of mental illness and temporary psychological abnormalities. Along with differences in temporal duration, mental disabilities differed in intensity, with incurable conditions like dementia praecox (now usually called schizophrenia) falling on the severe end of the spectrum and those like neurasthenia being classified as relatively mild. In order to account for a spectrum of mental illness, Katayama suggested that the Ministry of Justice use the term *seishin shōgai*, or mental disability, to refer to madness and include provisions in the law for the "limited responsibility" of offenders, rather than declare the existence or nonexistence of a crime. "There must be a clause (*ron*) about diminished responsibility," he wrote in a proposal to the committee charged with revisions, because it was impossible to clearly differentiate between someone with a healthy and a sick mind.

Arguing for a gradation theory was crucial to Katayama's interest in securing the authority of his new profession, for it was only specialists who could arguably distinguish for the court where the defendants fell on the spectrum of madness. Katayama gave a lecture in 1899 in which he explained:

[T]here are many kinds of mental illnesses (*seishinbyō*). First, there are ordinary people who, when examined, have mental illness. Second, there are times when a person appears to be mentally ill but in fact is not. Third, to a layperson it may appear that there is no abnormality of the mind when in fact a person is mentally ill. Fourth, there is the half-mad person, who is neither absolutely mentally ill nor entirely healthy-minded.

In the last case, Katayama argued that the punishment should be lessened.[13] Along with Katayama, other psychiatrists like Sakaki Hajime had all along argued that it was difficult to draw a clear boundary line between the sane and the mad. This is where Katayama located the authority and purpose of the *kantei*, or psychiatric evaluation. Because there was no clear line between sanity and insanity, an expert's opinion was required. Katayama was calling for psychiatric medicine to lead the law in reaching a just verdict and punishment.

Katayama faced considerable opposition from legal scholars regarding the inclusion of the medical concept of mental disability in the Criminal Code. Particularly vocal in his opposition to this medical term was Diet member and lawyer Hanai Takuzō who called for the phrase to be revised as "loss of heart and mind" (*shinshin sōshitsu*) to match the language used to describe the mentally incompetent in the Civil Code. Legal scholar Hozumi Nobushige agreed with Hanai and drew on Kure Shūzō's works to argue that "the phrase 'mental disability' also encompasses various kinds of meanings" and that in the end the meaning of the insanity clause "cannot possibly be said to be described [solely] by medical terminology."[14] Hozumi argued that there was no need for the insanity defense clause to take into consideration different types of mental illness. Tomi'i Masa'akira, a member of the House of Peers, also preferred that the language of Article 39 match that of the Civil Code. One historian has suggested that Tomi'i was wary of entrusting the determination of punishment to psychiatrists and other forensic doctors employed by the courts.[15] In the end, members of the Diet did not use Katayama's term "mental disability," but did incorporate his suggestion about accounting for diminished responsibility. Article 39 of the new Criminal Code promulgated in 1907 thus stated: "1) an incompetent person (literally, "a person who has lost his mind") shall not be punished; 2) a person with diminished competence (literally, "a person whose mind and body are diminished and weakened") shall receive a mitigation of punishment."[16]

Lawyers, legal scholars, and some politicians may have succeeded in implementing legal rather than psychiatric terminology in the Criminal Code of 1907, but psychiatrists and others in their camp continued to argue for a privileged place for their professional expertise. As Kure wrote in regard to the distinction made between a person who has "lost" his mind and one whose "mind and body are diminished and weakened" in the 1907 revision, "even if we [psychiatrists] try to interpret this, it does not accord with the actual conditions of mental disability, [making] it almost impossible to put in practice. It is therefore necessary to consult a psychiatrist to determine an explanation of these two kinds of persons."[17] In a nearly self-contradictory statement, Kure declared that the wording in the Criminal Code of 1907 did not reflect "actual" experiences of madness, as captured in the psychiatric term "mental disability," so a psychiatrist must be expected to clarify whether a defendant had suffered from either a "loss" or a "weakening" of the mind.

Yet for the psychiatric profession to take on the task of making such determinations in the context of criminal court cases, it would need further institutionalization and state support. As Yamane Masatsugu, a member of House of Representatives, stated in a proposition submitted to the Diet in 1906, the law existed but there were not enough qualified psychiatrists to perform the role of expert witness:

> In imperial Japan, although there is a provision for the legal punishment of a mentally ill patient (*seishinbyō kanja*) in the civil and criminal codes, in the public and private medical schools that ought to be training the doctors assigned to perform the [court-ordered] examinations for mental illness, there are absolutely no appropriate facilities necessary for the research [on mental illness]. Furthermore, the discipline of psychiatry (*seishinbyō gakka*) does not appear under the subjects covered by the medical license examination of the Ministry of Education, which assesses the qualifications of general practitioners. As a result, in practice, the nation is not only unable to interpret an important [part] of the law but [it is also] a great [source of] unhappiness for mentally ill persons as well as for ordinary citizen-subjects.[18]

In his opening remarks to the Diet, Yamane emphasized that "there are very few physicians who can diagnose mental illness in imperial Japan," which he saw as a "great shortcoming." He called for an examination in psychiatry, arguing that the state ought to add psychiatry to the general qualifications medical examination and fund the creation of psychiatry departments and research facilities inside medical schools. The reasons for such expansion, he claims, were twofold: to meet the standards of medical progress of other "civilized countries" and to establish a fully functioning legal system. As Yamane's demands in the Diet suggest, psychiatry had not acquired a recognized place even within the medical sciences, let alone law. Outside the halls of science, psychiatric concepts became better known once they found platforms through other disciplines and discourses, especially ones concerning gender and crime.

Female Crime in the Popular Imagination

Vocabularies of madness concerning female crime mixed and mingled across such disciplines as psychiatry, criminology, and sexology in an array of genres of popular culture in the early twentieth century. Popular notions of the inner (mis)workings of women's minds and bodies had deep roots in previous centuries. Mental and emotional disorders like menstrual psychosis were, to some extent, new formulations of old prejudices against women, repackaging Edo rhetoric about the unreliability and emotional volatility of women in an updated language of psychological and social pathology. In Kaibara Ekken's *Onna daigaku* (Greater Learning for Women, 1672), a manual of ethics and proper behavior for women of the samurai class, Ekken expressed widely shared views of women as inferior to men and afflicted by the five infirmities of indocility, discontent, slander, jealousy, and silliness. He pronounced that "female genitalia, while necessary for the reproduction of male heirs, were linked to dull-wittedness, laziness, lasciviousness, a hot temper, and a tremendous capacity to bear grudges."[19] The popular discourse on female psychological instability in the early twentieth century drew on older, neo-Confucian discourse about women's physical and mental inferiority to men.

The link between female physiology and crime, too, was made long before the appearance of the menstrual psychosis defense in the criminal courts of the early twentieth century. In the Edo period, officials frequently justified mitigated sentences for petty crime by a woman, noting that she was menstruating or pregnant and hence could not be held entirely responsible for her actions.[20] This kind of biocentric explanation, which interpreted social discord as the result of physiological and mental deviance, appeared in the figure of the "poison woman" (*dokufu*) in the 1870s. The poison woman first appeared as sensational temptress in Japan's first serialized novels, and thereafter traveled to other mass press sources such as kabuki plays, woodblock-printed books, memoirs, and short stories. The term referred to women who had committed sensational (and sensationalized) crimes of murder, robbery, or both. The crimes of the twenty female criminals labeled "poison women" in the late nineteenth century were attributed to their sexual behavior and bodily comportment, diverting attention from the possible social or psychological motives for committing them.

One of the best-known poison women, Takahashi Oden, called "Demon" Oden, was beheaded in 1879 for the murder of Gōtō Kichizō, a merchant in the Nihonbashi neighborhood of Tokyo. In serialized newspaper stories and woodblock-print books, both fictional and nonfictional, Oden's crime was attributed to her sexual deviance. Kanagaki Robun's *Takahashi Oden yasha monogatari* (The Tale of Demon Takahashi Oden) (1879) emphasized Oden's sexual aberrations through illustrative drawings of an autopsy. Oden's physical abnormalities supposedly provided proof of an unusual, excessive sexual energy that produced criminal behavior. Into the 1930s, somatic analyses of female deviants were discussed with little reference to ideological or social concerns. As literary scholar Christine Marran has shown, "a long-lived popular science that sought to explain crime by women via the body" originated with the treatment of women like Oden, whose "reproductive organs were preserved in formaldehyde by the original doctor presiding over the 1879 autopsy and passed from research collection to research collection to be once again analyzed in 1935 (!)."[21]

Unique to the early twentieth century was the rise of the "science of crime" (*hanzai kagaku*), or criminology, which provided new scientific and institutional support for an old argument about female criminality. The discipline of criminology was informed by a range of other new sciences spreading around the world, including sexology, psychiatry, psychology, and psychoanalysis.[22] Interest in crime flourished among Japanese scholars and the general public alike, as suggested by the sharp rise in the establishment of medical organizations and local clubs devoted to criminology. The Japanese Association of Criminology, founded in 1913, was composed of specialists from fields like psychology, psychiatry, legal medicine, law, and sociology. During the "textual crime wave" of the 1920s when scores of criminology journals and encyclopedias were published, the association announced in its own publication the following statement: "The mission of this magazine is to expose the secrets of the human instinct that produces all social ills and social goods, and to investigate thoroughly all aspects of human sciences. This magazine over the ensuing years will do all that it can to produce an encyclopedia that will gather resources on criminality, the scientific, and the bizarre." The journal claimed to bring to the Japanese public a transformation already occurring in Western Europe and the United States, namely a shift "from the pursuit of mechanical science to the mind sciences (*seishin kagaku*)."[23]

The impact of Euro-American discourse on the formation of Japanese criminology is undisputable. One might assume that the works of Italian criminologist Cesare Lombroso had a significant impact, as they did elsewhere. Lombroso's theory of the "born criminal," which argued that criminals were characterized by certain physical characteristics (such as a receding forehead and handle-shaped ears) that marked them as a distinct anthropological type, had prompted the establishment of criminology as a field of knowledge in many parts of Europe and the United States.[24] But as in the case of psychiatry, criminology in Japan before World War I was most influenced by German criminology, which tended to reject Lombroso's anthropological model and instead promote "criminal biology," or theories that stressed biological and psychological causes of crime.[25] The dominant figures in German criminology showed little interest in physical defects and focused instead on mental deficiencies, primarily "imbecility" and "lack of resilience." Criminal psychologist Gustav Aschaffenburg, for instance, referred to these mental conditions as "mental abnormalities" or "personality disorders" situated in the borderland between mental health and mental illness.

Another crucial influence was German jurist Franz von Liszt's theories of criminal law, which prompted Japanese legal scholars and jurists to incorporate notions of the individual and individuality into their new legal system. Liszt and his fellow reformers argued that the purpose of punishment was not retribution, but the prevention of individual criminals from committing offenses again in the future. They proposed that an offender's punishment should therefore depend not on the offense itself, but the potential dangerousness of the individual. As a result, German criminologists became interested in the person of the criminal and in the causes of criminal behavior.[26] How might one assess an offender's dangerousness? What kind of treatment would effectively help prevent an individual from committing a crime again? Legal scholar Makino Eiichi, who studied under Liszt at the University of Berlin in 1910, became the main proponent of this approach to criminal law in Japan, arguing that individual personality and lifestyle influenced his or her actions. "The essence (*honshitsu*) of crime," he wrote, "does not lie in the offense but in the offender."[27] Psychiatrists interested in crime, like Sugie Tadasu, adopted Makino's theories to identify personality and individuality (*kojinsei*) as the driving forces behind crime. Who people were in an ontological sense, and not their actions, were deemed pathological, and their dangerousness, or threat to public security and peace, stemmed from their potential to commit future crimes.

The new discipline of criminology gained traction in the 1920s and 1930s because of domestic factors, too. The booming interest in crime can be explained, in part, by an actual increase in the crime rate beginning in the mid-1920s. Once the prosperity following World War I dissipated and economic recession hit in 1924, aggravated by the great earthquake that struck Tokyo and Yokohama in September 1923, the crime rate increased steadily. The number of Criminal Code offenses brought to the Public Prosecutor's Office increased from 298,525 in 1920 to 545,360 in 1934. The number of reported thefts rose from 13,121 in 1920 to 16,508 in 1930, and the number of people convicted of crimes increased from 137,804 in 1920 to 163,192 in 1930. Most criminologists attributed the rise in crime mainly to poverty in rural, farming areas and to increased unemployment in the cities.[28]

Alongside such figures, concerns about the menace of crime escalated as social reformers and cultural critics once again lamented the arrival of a time of moral decadence and social transgression with the economic recession of the late 1920s. In the wake of the global stock market crash in 1929, poverty and communist-driven revolts created a charged political and cultural atmosphere. A growing popular phenomenon known as "erotic grotesque nonsense" generated a sensibility that reveled in science, sex, the occult, the foreign, and the bizarre, which also helped to spread criminological discourse in the popular media. In crime thrillers and detective fiction written by Edogawa Rampo and Yumeno Kyūsaku, the erotic-perverse drawings and prints of Itō Seiu, and other such works, theories linking women's crimes with their bodies and sexuality found fertile ground in which to flourish.[29]

Japanese criminologists, especially those versed in current theories of sexology and psychiatry, championed a biocentric discourse that connected women's physiological makeup to their tendency to commit crime.[30] Habuto Eiji and Sawada Junjirō, among the first working in the fields of sexology and criminology to formulate theories about women and crime, wrote in their 1916 *Research on Crime* (Hanzai no kenkyū) that the tendency to commit crimes caused by physiological makeup was greater for women than for men because their "reproductive functions are much more complicated than men's." There was therefore "a greater chance that [these reproductive functions] will have a damaging effect on mental faculties with the result that crimes brought on by the reproductive functions in women are considerable."[31] Such reproductive functions included puberty, menstruation, pregnancy, and menopause.

Menstruation had long been simultaneously celebrated and stigmatized in Japan. On the one hand, it was seen as a sacred, physical sign of coming of age, commemorated with special religious and communal rituals in some parts of the country. On the other hand, menstruation was considered a source of pollution, generating a culture of menstrual taboo informed in part by Buddhist ideas of defilement that prevented menstruating women from participating in various court and religious rituals from the tenth century on. Villagers in some regions of Japan built menstrual huts (*tabigoya*) to segregate women during their menstrual cycles.

Menstruation acquired new political meanings in the context of nation-building and rapid industrialization of the late nineteenth century. As an indicator of women's potential to procreate and help build a strong and powerful nation of healthy citizen-subjects, the issue of menstruation became a part of "motherhood protection" (*bosei hogo*) campaigns that argued for the necessity of measures such as "menstrual leave" for female factory workers.[32]

Yet, as suggested by the rise of new medical diagnoses such as menstrual psychosis, menstruation was also seen as a potential source of pathological and socially deviant behavior. Either of value or of danger, menstruation occupied an equivocal place in a polarizing discourse on women's bodies and sexuality.

At the height of the criminology boom in the late 1920s, popular and specialist publications featured studies of the association of women and crime. The sixteen-volume *Modern Criminology* series (*Kindai hanzai kagaku*) began publication in 1929, for instance, with four of its volumes covering women and crime. In one of them, *The Criminal Psychology* (*Hanzaisha no shinri*, 1930), psychiatrist Kaneko Junji argued that crime rates for women increased dramatically during menstruation and other reproductive functions including pregnancy: "Of course the onset of menses is a physiological function in which the lining of the womb is expelled within five days or so, but if we hypothesize that menstruation were to continue every day, and calculate the criminal danger of that menstrual cycle, we would find that the female crime rate would near that of the male crime rate."[33] All the more reason, Kaneko seems to imply, that one ought to be grateful that women did not menstruate every day. In the opening lines of another volume in the series, *Women and Crime* (*Josei to hanzai*, 1930), Nozoe Atsuyoshi wrote:

> The psychology of women's crimes is intimately connected to the physiological influences of women's bodies. And that there is a difference in the role played by men's sexual desires versus women's sexual desires in the committing of crimes is so obvious that there is no need to repeat it again here. For women, there is something that triggers a kind of revolution in the spiritual-psychological life of a young girl, and it is called menstruation (*gekkei*).[34]

After establishing the primacy of menstruation, Nozoe goes on to argue that crime by heterosexual men was not hormonal but intellectual in origin. Men committed crimes as a result of their protracted struggle in the social world. The pressures of nation-building and capitalist growth in which they participated led them to commit crimes because they were progressive and mentally charged. Women, on the other hand, followed their instincts uncontrollably: "Women's relationship to nature is more primitive than that of men. They have a less developed constitution; consequently, their innate instincts operate more freely. Just as the instinct for cruelty is common in the animal world, this erupts more easily and more dramatically than in men."[35]

By the 1930s, the connection between crime and menstruation was widely invoked in popular discourse. As politician Katayama Tetsu, who became prime minister in 1947, commented in an issue of *Women's Review* (*Fujin kōron*): "When do women commit the most crimes? When are there the most fires and accidents triggered by the ill-caution of women? There's no need to ask these questions of expert physicians, for it is common knowledge today—everyone agrees that it is during times of menstruation."[36] Yet popular and expert consensus notwithstanding, some of the same publications that featured male doctors and criminologists reinforcing patriarchal gender norms offered women's own narratives, too. Drawing from forensic psychiatric reports and other court documents, some publications documented the ways in which women on trial for crimes expressed their interests, needs, and motivations in ways that complicated—if not defied—expert testimonies about women's minds and bodies. The narratives of crime offered by the women on trial reveal the limitations and reductive quality of the biocentric discourse that attributed women's crime to the inner workings of their bodies. In doing so, the narratives provide the social and individual context missing from explanations focused solely on female reproductive processes, as well as a sense of a vernacular language of "bloody inversion" with which women made sense of their bodies and behaviors.

Interviews with Women in Forensic Psychiatric Reports

Although Japanese criminal court records from the first half of the twentieth century are notoriously difficult to find, one compelling documentary source of women's own explanations of their crimes exists in the form of a medical and legal document known as a "mental evaluation" (*seishin kantei*), or forensic psychiatric report. Written by psychiatrists and physicians serving as expert witnesses in criminal cases, the forensic psychiatric reports provided psychiatric-medical assessments of the defendant's mental state before, during, and after her crime. The examining psychiatrist would weave together information garnered from physical examinations, interviews with the defendant as well as her family and acquaintances, and police or trial documents in order to fashion a narrative that could help determine the extent of the defendant's responsibility for the crime. Although the women's stories were highly mediated by the voice of the examining psychiatrist, these reports still prove an invaluable source of the defendants' points of view.

In Japan, the forensic psychiatric report was formally introduced in 1895 with the publication of the first translation of a textbook of forensic psychiatry, literally "judiciary mental medical science" (*shihō seishin igaku*): psychiatrists Kure Shūzō and Katayama Kunika's translation of Austrian psychiatrist Eduard R. von Hofmann's *Lehrbuch der gerichtlichen Medicin*.[37] The first Japanese forensic psychiatric textbook was published two years later by Kure and Sakaki Hajime.[38] Even before the publication of these textbooks, psychiatrists and physicians were conducting mental assessments of defendants, the first in 1882 for the trial of a woman accused of murdering her child.[39] There are two main collections of forensic psychiatric reports, compiled by the examining psychiatrists themselves in the late nineteenth century: Sakaki Hajime's *Seishin jōkyō kantei shoshū*, which contained reports submitted for civil cases from 1887 to 1896; and Kure Shūzō's compendia of published reports of forty-five criminal cases.[40]

Neither the law nor the medical profession provided a standardized format for the forensic psychiatric reports submitted to civil and criminal courts, but the reports tended to be similarly organized. Most began with a brief description of the details of the case—the sequence or time and place of the crime—and the defendant's biographical information, including her past medical history, childhood upbringing, and family medical history (*idenreki*). In the physician's interview of the defendant about her medical history, he asked about the beginning of puberty and when she started to menstruate, and about her mood or behavior during menstruation. The report would then turn to present-day symptoms. The examining psychiatrist or physician would often conduct a physical examination of the defendant and report the results of her hearing, eyesight, and more, followed by excerpts from the oral interviews conducted with the defendant as part of sections called "psychological symptoms" (*seishin shōjō*). These excerpts were usually taken verbatim from the transcripts of interviews and were supposed to convey to readers the defendant's own words and explanations to questions ranging from "do you know why you are here today?" to "how do you feel at that time of the month?" The forensic psychiatric report would then conclude with a seemingly definitive explanation by the examining physician in which he would make a final diagnosis about the state of mind of the defendant before, during, and after the crime.

The forensic report was organized as a search for an answer to the question of whether the defendant suffered from a mental illness that might relieve her of responsibility for her crime. It was not intended as an assessment of the extent of her responsibility, but rather as an expert medical report on her mental state. As psychiatrist Sugie Tadasu wrote in a section on the purpose and format of a psychiatric forensic report in a compendium of books on the topic of medical jurisprudence (*hōigaku*), or "legal medicine," in 1897, "whether [the defendant] is responsible (*sekinin nōryoku*) or not, ought to be punished or not, is not for the medical physician to make a statement. [His] only [concern] is to judge the health or diseased state of the mind (*seishin*) in accordance with scientific examination procedures."[41] The author of forensic psychiatric reports, often psychiatrists but also general physicians, narrated their findings to maximize suspense. The reports presented clues to induce the reader to surmise what the result might be, evoking similarities with the plots of mysteries and crime thrillers popular in the 1920s.[42] The examining physician likely arranged and selected information to include in the first part of the report—all the factual details, including the words of the defendant—in ways that rendered the final diagnosis scientific, logical, and even inevitable.

The forensic psychiatric report thus contained a double narrative: the defendant's story was embedded and retold in the psychiatrist's scientific and official account. The medical story was a redaction of the defendant's earlier presentation. Embedded in the medical narrative were the voices and words of other people, including the defendant's family and other witnesses to the case. The report consisted of layers of narrative that turned an individual physician's interpretation of the patient's subjective and private experience of both illness and crime into a seemingly objective, scientific—or reliably inter-subjective and medically recognizable—account of disease.[43] Yet the remarks of defendants and witnesses did not always conform to the logic and rhetoric of the expert witness. It thus becomes possible to catch glimpses of such remarks that disrupt even the most seemingly coherent psychiatric witness account.

Glimpses of the words and worlds of female defendants appear in such publications as *Hōigaku tanpenshū* [Collected Stories of Medical Jurisprudence, 1930]. A volume of a well-known criminology series, *Hōigaku tanpenshū* featured a series of redactions of forensic psychiatric reports submitted to Kyoto district courts in the 1910s and 1920s.[44] The redactions consisted of composites of medical examinations, legal documents, and confessional interviews, with many parts censored for privacy reasons, all conducted in the context of determining verdicts for female defendants. Edited by Takada Giichirō, a physician, writer, criminologist, and sexologist, the volume would have appealed to a broad audience of specialists and popular readers alike. When read alongside other forensic reports and newspaper reports of more famous cases of female crime in the same time period, it is possible to discern parts of the broader cultural script about women's bodily malfunctions being invoked but also contested by female defendants.

In a case of "temporary insanity" in the 1920s, the attempted arson of a housewife named "Ita" (full name censored) is represented in a forensic psychiatric report as having occurred in the context of strained familial relations and resentment. Arson had long been considered a serious crime. Since the Edo period, arson, especially in densely populated and wooded metropolises like Edo, Kyoto, and Osaka, was a crime treated with severe forms of punishment, including burning at the stake and beheading. But even in the eighteenth century, suspects of arson deemed mentally deficient tended to receive lenient punishments, as shogunal officials took into account the convicted arsonist's mental condition.[45] In Ita's case, the attempted arson occurred within a domestic context. Around 4:30 on the morning of June 13, Ita woke up unusually early, washed her face, and stepped outside. She walked over to her neighbor's house, where she saw bags of charcoal under the eaves. She then set fire to it, without consciously understanding her motivation. She claimed that she simply "flared up" (*noboseru*) because she was menstruating:

ITA: My ten-year-old child is mute, and [my neighbor, who is also my cousin] says mean things about her . . . (cries) . . . I had spent the day [before the crime] crying. And when I woke up in the morning (cries) I had gotten my period, and I flared up too much (*yokeini nobosete*) and thoughtlessly. . . .
PHYSICIAN: What month was that?
ITA: June 13th. I stood near the eaves [of my neighbor's house], where there were three pine trees and two sacks of charcoal, which I lit on fire.
PHYSICIAN: Why?
ITA: I don't really understand myself. I just flared up and did it.
PHYSICIAN: Are you like that normally?
ITA: I am usually fine but when my period arrives, I flare up.[46]

In just this brief excerpt, Ita used three variations of the expression *noboseru* (or *gyakujō suru*), which literally means "up into reverse" and is translated here as "flare up." Many female defendants invoked this expression in order to explain what happened to their minds and bodies when they were menstruating. The expression appeared in a wide range of print and media sources in the nineteenth and early twentieth centuries, from kabuki plays and political novels to philosophical tracts, in reference to a physical and emotional state in which blood flowed upward to the head, triggering a state of excitability that usually led to mental instability. Echoing pre-nineteenth-century medical and cultural ideas of the mind and body as constituted by flows of *ki* energy, the term evoked the notion of an imbalance and irregular flow of energy in the form of blood. One popular hygiene manual from 1908 defined the term as the state in which "blood washes up excessively to the brain." Women were not exclusively affected. Late nineteenth-century newspaper accounts describe male rickshaw drivers and inn owners whose "flare-ups" led to various forms of mad or strange behavior. The term was thus associated with the "enflamed" passionate states of mind among both men and women prior to the commitment of such grave crimes as murder and arson.[47] Yet when women on trial in the 1920s and early 1930s used such phrases, they specifically evoked images of the flowing of blood not only to the head but out of their bodies in the form of menstruation. Women closely associated "flare-ups" with menstruation and what some now call menopause. When asked by court-hired physicians how they felt while menstruating, many female defendants described their "flare-ups." Examining physicians and psychiatrists, too, deployed the term to describe the states of body and mind of the female defendants, acknowledging its broad circulation.

Another related term that was used by both female defendants and their families was *kan*, as in the phrase "*kan ga tatte*," or literally, "nerves stand up." Rather than use the language of nerves introduced through European medical texts in the nineteenth century, they invoked *kan* with its deep roots in a Sino-Japanese medical and cultural model of the mind and body. The term underwent a shift in meaning and use in the Edo period from a descriptor for the loss of consciousness and foaming at the mouth to a more comprehensive concept that covered such symptoms and conditions as "fright," "seizure," and "madness." *Kan* was considered to be particularly common among women, causing uneasy sleep, nightmares, stuffiness in the chest, dizziness, headache, and more. In some instances, it was considered as the source of "madness in women" and "women's blood-related diseases," alongside "depression, anger, regret, frustration, worry, uneasiness, fright, flushing, and headache."[48] Into the early twentieth century, advertisements for patent medicines that treated women's diseases often simply described the product as "effective in curing *kan*."

In the case of attempted arson by the female defendant Ita, the examining physician further contextualized her descriptions of "flaring up" in strained relations within her extended family. The defendant had been twenty-two years old when she married her husband, with whom she had a son and two daughters. One daughter died prematurely and the eldest daughter was "mute" and "dim-witted" (*gudon*), so the defendant was very worried about her. Her neighbor, who happened to be her cousin, not only said "mean things" about the defendant's "mute" daughter but also suspected the defendant once when some money went missing, which the defendant had found "extremely disagreeable." When the defendant was arrested by the police, she confessed to having committed the crime of arson and, in that moment, to use the psychiatrist's summation, "a great deal of menstrual blood flowed out, and so there was the suspicion that this arson was related to her menstruation."[49] When asked about the suspected theft, Ita responded in the following way:

PHYSICIAN: What about the 20 yen from [your cousin's] house?
ITA: That has nothing to do with me. I don't know anything about that.
PHYSICIAN: Were you angry that she had said mean things about [your mute daughter]?
ITA: It lingered in my heart somewhat.
PHYSICIAN: Were relations bad between you two?
ITA: No, it wasn't bad. I just suddenly flared up.
PHYSICIAN: Did you really set the fire?
ITA: Ummm yes, I was the one who started the fire. Although the prosecutor told me that if it wasn't me then I should say so, I was, indeed, the one who lit the match.[50]

The examining physician was willing to consider the role of Ita's prior resentment toward her cousin and the stress of raising a disabled daughter, but in the end, he concluded that Ita's menstruation, and not the domain of kinship, was the key to explaining her crime.

How might Ita and other female defendants have known that it could be to their benefit to employ the language of "flaring up" to suggest that they were not in control of their mind or behavior due to their menses? During Ita's preliminary hearing, the prosecutor or judge asked specific questions about her menstruation, such as "Do your hands and feet get numb when you are menstruating?" and "Has there ever been a time when you were bothersome to others while you were menstruating?" Like other women on trial for crimes at this time, Ita responded by saying that yes, her mood was linked to her menstrual cycle, that she would feel "on edge" (*musha kusha*) and "flare up" (*noboseru*) when she had her period. The preliminary hearing may have been the first place where she learned to use this language, but this wording was already in wide circulation in everyday discourse to describe women's moods during their menstrual cycles. The link made by medical physicians and criminologists between menstruation and crime would have also been an idea broadly enough circulated that some female defendants spoke openly about how she and other women in the family bonded over how "it is easy for women to flare up to an extreme" while they were both admitted into Ōji Brain Hospital for mental disturbance.[51]

Women clearly understood the examining psychiatrist's intention to try to link their crimes with their menstruation cycles. A woman named "Fu" (full name censored), also accused of arson, responded in the following way when prompted during a second session with an examining physician to speak about their previous session:

PHYSICIAN: When did you last see me?
FU: September.
PHYSICIAN: What did we talk about then?
FU: You asked me various things about my sexual desires. Then we talked about my menstruation and my brothers and sisters.
PHYSICIAN: What day is it today?
FU: The 27th.
PHYSICIAN: Do you know who I am?
FU: You are the person who will from now on ask about things like the times I have my period and how [I started a fire] because of my bodily [functions].
PHYSICIAN: What is my occupation?
FU: You're a doctor (isha).[52]

Fu then explained that around the time that she was sent to be a servant in another household, her brother was hospitalized for gonorrheal ophthalmia. Upset about her brother's illness and her mother's consequent anxiety about his condition, Fu grew increasingly resentful of the household in which she was newly hired. Then the thought arose of setting fire to it to make it disappear: "I went to the bathroom, lit the fire. It was around 3 in the morning. But the patrolmen came. I regret doing it." At first, the family asked Fu if she knew who did it. She hesitated at first, intending to lie, but then told the truth to the patrolmen. At no point in the forensic psychiatric report does Fu refer to menstruation as having played a role in her behavior and activities; she understands her crime as having occurred within the domain of kinship. Her case suggests that women understood their bodies and behaviors as intimately connected to the stresses and pressures of the precarious lives of the lower class, most of whom had little medical recourse when they or their families were afflicted by ill health and remained at the mercy of their employers.

Women's crimes often occurred within intimate and institutional contexts that involved sexual violence, as in the complicated case of arson in 1924 involving a divorcee-turned-Buddhist nun in her mid-twenties named "Kai" (full name censored). The examining physician was clearly captivated by this woman. He described her as an alluringly "feminine" and yet bold woman:

> The defendant's figure is enticing (*namamekashii*) and her movements are feminine (*onna rashiku*). She is verbose in conversation, and she always smiles or laughs loudly during the examinations. She is well dressed, and comes to each examination after having changed [her attire]. In her interactions with people she remains quite undaunted, without the appearance of modesty. She talks nonchalantly about things that a woman would typically find embarrassing. Her facial expressions are lively.[53]

In the physician's eyes, Kai simultaneously played the role of a coquettish, feminine woman who had a mind of her own, talking nonchalantly about things that most women, he assumed, would find embarrassing, presumably topics such as her menstrual cycle and sexual experiences. The forensic psychiatric report affirmed this representation of Kai. Her own words, too, suggest intolerance for certain social expectations that had accumulated through the years.

Born in Nagoya to a working-class family in the tobacco manufacturing industry, Kai moved with her parents to Tokyo when she was three years old. There her family ran an unsuccessful antique store. The psychiatrist describes her as having been raised "in the manner of *shita-machi*" because her family resided in the plebeian neighborhood of Tsukiji. When she was eighteen years old, she was "solicited" by her younger brother's painting instructor and was soon married off to the second son in the same family of the name "Oki" (full name censored). The Oki household was one of high standing, having accumulated wealth through "business affairs," but because Kai's family was relatively poor, she did not bring much money with her. Although she lived in a household with an older sister-in-law as well as two middle-aged sisters-in-law, Kai suffered emotionally and was overworked, so much so that it induced an "abnormality in the mind (*seishin ni ijō*)," in the psychiatrist's words. When her plan to commit suicide by throwing herself in the well was discovered, the family admitted her into Ōji Brain Hospital in Tokyo, where she was diagnosed with manic–depressive disorder (*sōutsushō*). Treated with bathing therapy, she gradually convalesced and left the hospital after about a month.

Back at home, Kai continued to suffer because she was treated so differently from her sisters-in-law and because, as the psychiatrist writes, "her husband was spineless (*ikuji no nai*)" and unable to defend his wife. In the end, Kai divorced her husband and left the household at age twenty-one.

At age twenty-three, Kai passed an entrance exam for a vocational school in Kanagawa prefecture. But deciding that she was interested in philosophy and religion, with the idea of attaining enlightenment, she went to Kamakura, a center of Buddhism. There she fell in love with "Man X" and then was raped by a "violent man" (*ranbōsha*), "Man Y," which prompted her to leave Kamakura. Without consulting her parents, she decided to shave her head and become a monk. So she left for Kyoto, where she found lodging in the Buddhist temple Kenninji, which was where she committed her crime of arson.

The turning point in Kai's life, according to the men whose statements appeared in this forensic report, was around the time of her hospitalization and divorce. Her father claimed in his deposition that "her personality changed completely after she was discharged from the hospital. Before she had been an extremely obedient woman. Once she came back from the hospital, she would easily fly into a rage, made excuses often, and expressed a desire to study."[54] In similar witness statements, one acquaintance described Kai as "a person whose mood changes easily. You would think she is living her life as a nun, but then she will say something like, perhaps I will start an inn. She is as fickle as a cat's eyes. When you see her she seems gentle but she is actually quite prideful and thinks that everyone else is stupid and she herself is superior."[55] Others described her as having "a high degree of hysteria" and "abnormalities of the mind" (*seishin no ijō*). Kai admitted that she committed arson:

PHYSICIAN: When did you commit the crime?
KAI: September 27.
PHYSICIAN: Did you really commit arson?
KAI: Yes, I did.
PHYSICIAN: Did you do so because you felt extremely distressed?

Her answer to this question was long, as she explained the romantic entanglements that got her into trouble at the Buddhist temple in Kyoto. Rumors had started to spread about a Buddhist priest named "Fuji" (full name censored), who had been seen walking around in a *yukata*, an informal summer kimono, implying that he had taken off his priestly garments and been seeking sexual pleasures. People seemed to have started talking about Kai and Fuji. The high priest of the temple decided to kick Fuji out because of these rumors. When Fuji came to tell Kai about this, Kai demanded that he better refute the rumors about the two of them before he left. "I also told him," Kai related, "not to come to my place anymore, but he refused. Others started to look at me with scornful eyes and I couldn't stand it!"[56]

The psychiatrist concluded that Kai, in late September 1924, was already experiencing manic–depressive disorder and had an excitable personality (*taishitsusei kōfunsha*). In part because of a dispute with the head priest of the temple concerning matters related to Fuji, and in part because of her own dissatisfaction with her spiritual practice, her mind had been over-wrought. Moreover, on October 1, she got her period, so on September 29, the defendant's mind had most certainly had various "abnormalities" (*ijō*). Yet the act of arson was not committed on a whim. It was premeditated and she put "much passionate consideration" into it, according to the psychiatrist. The previous day she had bought and prepared the petroleum, considering when and where she should start the fire. In such preparations, the psychiatrist detected no "mental abnormality." On the day of the crime, she drizzled oil in a closet inside the temple, and even thought to put an old basket into the closet so that the fire would catch more readily. She lit and threw about five matches until the basket caught fire, and left the door ajar so that the fire would burn better. Afterward, she ran away to Ōtsu, but then called an acquaintance at the temple to see if it had caught fire or not. The psychiatrist thus concluded that the crime was premeditated and so Kai must be held responsible for her crime, even if her menstrual cycle had made her more susceptible to criminal impulses.

Kai did not benefit from a menstrual psychosis defense because she showed no regret. The examining psychiatrist claimed that, when women committed crimes as a result of their menstrual cycles, they did it without planning and felt regret afterward. But Kai's case was different. She had a definite motive. When asked by the psychiatrist whether she believed taking revenge and the arson was a bad thing, she replied, "Except for intending to die, I did not do anything bad, and yet people said bad things about me, so I think an act to this degree is not bad." Furthermore, Kai did not want to benefit from a menstrual psychosis defense:

> If I say I set fire unexpectedly, then the punishment is diminished, right? I am not thinking about the degree of my punishment, though. People are saying that what I did was the act of a mad person (*kyōjin*)

or the result of a mental abnormality due to menstruation (*gekkeiji no seishin ijō*), but if that is how [my act] is seen, my efforts over the past several years amount to nothing![57]

Although Kai did not specify what such an "effort" consisted of, one could reasonably assume that she was referring to her decisions to leave behind marriage and family to pursue first her studies and then spiritual cultivation. She implied that she wanted her arson to be seen as something with purpose, an expression of her will. When asked directly in court by the prosecutor, "Do you think that this crime has something to do with your menstruation?" Kai responded quickly: "No, I don't think that at all." Here Kai chose to emphasize her conscious decisions and actions, suggesting that some women resisted the dominant biocentric discourse, even at the risk of receiving a harsher sentence.

Kai was likely not the only woman to refuse to accept the menstrual psychosis defense, an explanation that robbed defendants of intention and will. In 1916, Kamichika Ichiko, a journalist for the *Tokyo nichi nichi* newspaper, went on trial for attempted murder. On November 9, Kamichika had stabbed the well-known anarchist Ōsugi Sakae at a teahouse in Kanagawa prefecture. She was, it turned out, one of his lovers, supposedly jealous that he had taken another lover. According to newspaper reprints of the trial records, the crime was allegedly motivated by jealousy but Kamichika herself claimed that the crime was "retaliation against Ōsugi for having toyed with my virtue."[58] She claimed that she would have committed the crime even if Ōsugi had not taken another lover. She herself never mentioned her menstrual cycle, nor did she suggest that she was acting in a state of diminished competence. But her lawyer, Suzuki Fujiya, argued otherwise: "Since the defendant at the time of the crime was in a state of 'diminished and weakened mind and body' due to her menses, there is sufficient reason to reduce her sentence."[59] Like Kai, Kamichika was convicted for her crime of attempted murder and sentenced to four years in prison.[60]

Divorcee-turned-Buddhist-nun Kai was hardly the only woman whose crime occurred against a background of sexual violence. One forensic psychiatric reports gave insight into defendants like "Tani" (full name censored), an uneducated and impoverished woman in her twenties tried for attempted murder sometime between 1921 and 1926.[61] The report, which included citations from the arrest report and witness testimony, stated that Tani was raped ("her virtue was forcibly blemished") by "Nosuke" (full name censored) while employed as his maid servant. Their relationship continued until she became pregnant when she was nineteen years old. When she told Nosuke about the pregnancy, he dismissed her, forcing her to become a geisha and wander around looking for work. She returned to her mother's home in Osaka to give birth, but the baby soon died and Tani was forced to look for work again. A few years passed before she returned to her former employer to ask for a loan so that she could repay a debt she had incurred many years ago to another man. Nosuke "toyed with her virtue" but in the end refused to lend her any money. Desperate and hopeless, Tani decided to commit suicide. She bought a small knife, and then visited Nosuke in Kyoto to make one final plea. He ignored her pleas and hit and kicked her, which made her so angry that she pulled out the knife and cut him near his collarbone. She then chased after him into the street, where a patrolman saw them and apprehended her.

Other than the examining physician or psychiatrist, many others involved in the arrest and trial offered their interpretations of the female defendant's moods and personality. The police asked Tani about her menstrual cycle in their initial interrogation after her arrest, for instance:

POLICE: When did you get your period?
TANI: It is late from 4 to 10 days each month, so I can't really say for sure.
POLICE: Right before and after your cycle, do you feel any different from usual?
TANI: I am usually short-tempered (*tanki*). I get angry easily and throw things that are nearby. Right before my period, I get even more short-tempered, and get frustrated by even the smallest thing.[62]

Witness testimony corroborated this account of her temperament and mood during her monthly cycles. When asked about her personality, the plaintiff Nosuke replied: "She's an extremely hysterical woman (*hisuterii no tsuyoi onna*) so she has an easily excitable personality." When asked about how he felt about having been wounded, he responded: "I feel responsible for the hurt inflicted on me since it was a product of ignoring the 'way of humanity.' Tani is but a woman (*onna no koto de aru*), and I don't bear any grudge against her. I hope she receives as light a sentence as possible."[63] Another character witness from the family testified that "she is very intelligent, but when she has her period she gets terrible stomach pains and for four or five days she is hysteric-like (*hisuterii teki*), though otherwise she has a timid personality." Of course, it is possible that the examining physician purposefully did not in-clude statements of witnesses who may have characterized Tani in ways other than "excitable" or "hysterical" while menstruating. Still, the forensic psychi-atric report evokes the ways in which a range of witnesses drawn from the defendant's circle of kin and acquaintances deployed a language of hysteria to reinforce normative understandings of female criminals as "prisoners" to the effects of their bodily and reproductive functions.

The ultimate medical diagnosis for Tani reflected the extent to which even the examining physician was constrained by a legal process that compelled expert witnesses to produce clear statements about the female defendant's mental state and capacities at the time of the crime. The examining physician concluded that Tani's was a case of "temporary insanity" (*ichijisei seishin ijō*), not premeditated attempted murder. It was only because she was menstruating that she lashed out at Nosuke with a knife. The official medical assessment consisted of the following two points:

1. At the time of examination, the defendant was "normal," in the everyday sense of the term, and under the terms of the Criminal Code is a person wholly responsible (*kanzen sekinin nōryoku sha*).
2. At the time of the crime (January 29 of this year, around 7 P.M.) as well as right before and after, the defendant was in a temporary state of emotional excitement (*kanjō kyōfun jōtai*) because she was about to begin her menstrual cycle. To use the terms of Article 39 from the Criminal Code, she was in a state of "diminished competence" (*shinshin mōjaku*).

The medical examiner argued for equivalence between the medical diagnosis of "temporary insanity" and the legal concept of "diminished competence," claiming that the defendant must be held responsible for the crime, but that a reduced sentence was justified. The verdict of Tani's trial remains unknown, as does the judicial interpretation of the diagnosis "temporary insanity" in her case, but in her example as well as others, it is possible to see incongruities between medical and legal discourses, as well as the ways in which those discourses were interwoven with a female defendant's own accounts of her body and crime in criminal proceedings.

The female defendants whose stories appeared in forensic psychiatric reports tended to belong to the lower-middle and lower classes. With their employment either changing frequently or remaining undefined, these women often found themselves in socially and economically precarious circumstances.[64] Many were victims of sexual violence, either by intimate partners or employers. Both Tani and Kamichika, for instance, struck against men who were in socially superior positions and who had wronged them. Tani had been raped and impregnated by her employer, who had fired her when he found out about the pregnancy. Her case illuminates the threats and acts of sexual violence in the homes in which domestic servants labored. By using the phrase "toyed with my virtue," Kamichika suggested that, even though relations had likely been consensual, she had been misled and taken advantage of. Exploited by men, both women seem to have turned to acts that would be criminalized, regardless of whether they were premeditated. Yet the judicial system did not take into account economic precarity and sexual violence. Menstruation- or other reproductive-function-induced "madness" was more legible and therefore more acceptable in the courts than structural inequalities and gendered violence.

The crimes of women from this group attracted a disproportionate amount of attention in the media, too. The most famous example is Abe Sada, a geisha who confessed in 1936 to murdering her lover Ishida Kichizō by asphyxiating him with the pink sash of her kimono and severing his penis from his body with a kitchen knife.[65] Abe's sexual proclivities and desires became the touchstone for explaining her crime. As outcasts who belonged to marginalized social groups, these underclass women and their crimes perhaps received relatively more public attention because they evoked the difficulties of "incorporating the underclass citizen into the purportedly democratizing national body" in the early twentieth century.[66] The crimes of this specific social group helped produce images of "the generic female criminal as uncivilized, antithetical to social progress, and an example of the disaster that uncontrolled female desire can wreak" in the 1920s and 1930s.

Even just the bits and pieces of the women's explanations of their crimes that surface in the forensic psychiatric reports contradict the notion of a "generic" female criminal or universal female desire, both of which circulated widely in criminological, sexological, psychiatric, and popular discourses. The reports offer a powerful sense of the complexities of gender relations, family life, and social conditions that affected female defendants, as well as the overlaying of vocabularies of madness invoked by a wide range of actors. Each participant in the legal proceedings was constrained to some extent. Medical expert witnesses may have been sympathetic to the women's plights, but what mattered in the context of the trial was for them to provide a medical diagnosis of the defendants' states of mind. Defense lawyers aimed to secure the most minimal punishment possible and thus deployed defenses of menstruation-induced temporary insanity sometimes against their client's wishes. The testimonies of the women suggest that their reactions varied. The menstrual psychosis defense was implicitly embraced by some of the women and rejected by others, like Kai, who tried to reclaim her agency in the crime committed by rejecting the possibility that a menstrual mood disorder or other form of mental illness drove her to arson. Kai thus rejected judicial leniency, which amounted to a criticism of the decriminalization of her acts. Defendants like Kai seem to have recognized that treating women as legally "irresponsible" as a result of the hysteria allegedly induced by their reproductive systems reinforced patriarchal, normative understandings of women's sexuality and gender roles in the family.

Yet such women's claims to autonomy occurred within narratives that highlighted the ways in which the same women's bodies and behaviors, whether declared criminal or not, were embedded within the domain of kinship. The fathers, mothers, intimate partners, domestic employers, and other kin who served as character witnesses are either implicitly or explicitly implicated in the embodied experiences of crime as caried out by the women on trial. The judicial process aimed to localize and isolate "criminal behavior" within the body of one woman, but the women on trial powerfully gestured toward such behavior originating outside of their bodies to some extent, and as part of a complex web of connected kin and relations.

Epilogue: Postwar Cultures of Gendered Care and Kinship

THE HISTORY OF family-based care for those considered mad and its effects on women in nineteenth- and twentieth-century Japan reveals some striking continuities across time. The family-centered cultures and structures of medico-religious healing of the Edo period did not disappear with the new Meiji regime's efforts in the 1870s and 1880s to remake the Japanese medical system so that it aligned with biomedical ones developing in Western Europe, the United States, and their colonies. Families continued to manage medico-religious care during a time of far-reaching social and geopolitical change. Government officials, intellectuals, psychiatrists, and others attempted to re-define fox-spirit attachment as "superstition" and "mental illness" beginning in the 1880s, but many families reported bouts of madness incited by fox spirits well into the twentieth century. Through the 1970s to 1990s, psychiatrists and folklorists would continue to conduct surveys, write case studies, and publish research on fox-spirit-attachment in rural villages.[1] Home confinement, too, persisted across the often-presumed divide between the Edo and Meiji periods in the mid-nineteenth century. Subject to intensified official scrutiny and police surveillance at the turn of the twentieth century, home confinement remained the most common form of management of those who were considered mad and prone to violence until the practice was banned in 1950.[2]

It would be a mistake to think that family-centered cultures and structures of care persisted because of the inherent power of long-standing ideas and practices. This book has shown that the centrality of family in the care of those considered mad endured because the state and its various supporters enforced and institutionalized it through law, ideology, and bureaucracy. The Meiji state created a series of laws, from the Household Registration laws in the

Madness in the Family. H. Yumi Kim, Oxford University Press. © Oxford University Press 2022.
DOI: 10.1093/oso/9780197507353.003.0006

1870s to the Civil Code of 1898 and the Custody Law of 1900, that required families to bear responsibility for their sick, mentally disturbed, or otherwise incapacitated members. It also refused to allocate enough resources to build a social welfare system or nationwide system of hospital-based care, even as psychiatrists criticized the legal and bureaucratic regulation of family-based care as insufficient and inhumane. With the family as the available default, there was little incentive for the state to create an alternative resource, especially at a time when the patriarchal family was being ideologically touted as a micro-version of a nation and empire, with an emperor-like father at its head.

At the same time, the Japanese legal system did not uniformly hold the family responsible for crimes committed by those suffering from madness across the twentieth century. As seen in cases of women in the 1920s and 1930s who committed violent crimes supposedly under the influence of their menstrual cycles, civil laws that outlined domestic responsibility had no traction in criminal trials. In a new criminal law system that no longer recognized collective entities like families as responsible for crime but instead held the individual accountable, the state was compelled to intervene. Professionals within the legal system would then both adjudicate and medically evaluate the behaviors of a mentally unstable person. Families played a role in legal proceedings as witnesses but could not be held legally responsible for the actions of their kin.

"Family responsibility" for those deemed mentally ill took on other meanings as Japan entered war, first with China and then the world from 1937 to 1945. This period witnessed the consolidation of the eugenics movement, which rendered families as sites of the transmission of traits considered undesirable in efforts to "improve the Japanese race." Calls for racial improvement had appeared as early as in the 1880s, first in the face of Western imperialist threats and then in building an empire in East Asia, but it was not until the 1920s and 1930s when reproductive issues among women were framed as "social problems" that eugenics discourse became widespread.[3] Promoters of eugenics attributed an array of "social problems" to heredity (*iden*), identifying conditions such as venereal disease, alcoholism, leprosy, intellectual disability, and mental illness as the main causes of "racial degeneration." They then called for measures such as marriage restrictions, quarantines, castration, sterilization, and birth control.[4] The wartime imperial state also claimed that mental illnesses such as schizophrenia and manic depression were hereditary, even as psychiatrists across the Japanese empire questioned the scientific accuracy of such a claim.[5] As a result, the first eugenics law in 1940 called for those with "hereditary mental illnesses" (*idensei seishinbyō*) to be sterilized.

But mass sterilization did not occur in the early 1940s, partly because most mentally ill persons were confined at home rather than hospitals. This made it difficult for the state and psychiatrists to adequately access patients and conduct sterilizations.[6] Mass sterilization became feasible only after World War II, when the legal and therapeutic landscape of madness shifted so dramatically that the role of family and kin, so crucial during the period covered in this book, seemed to disappear.

From Home to Hospital?

After World War II, a series of laws and financial incentives shifted structures of care such that hospitals replaced the home as the most common site of treatment for severe mental illnesses. During the Allied Occupation of Japan (1945–1952), the Ministry of Health and Welfare strove to implement a social welfare system that aligned with the postwar Constitution's goals of upholding the rights of citizens and safeguarding their health. In 1950, the Mental Hygiene Law replaced the Custody Law of 1900, making it illegal to confine mentally ill persons at home or any place other than a hospital.[7] Like the Mental Hospital Law of 1919, the Mental Hygiene Law called for the establishment of mental hospitals in each prefecture but, unlike its precedent, it required the state to bear half of the expenses of operating a psychiatric facility. The Ministry of Health and Welfare also recognized the shortage of psychiatric facilities in the country and provided loans for building private institutions, which, in a national context of rapid postwar economic growth, produced what was known as the "mental hospital boom." Many psychiatric hospitals were built during this boom, some with questionable credentials. Between 1954 and 1961, the number of psychiatric hospitals more than doubled from 224 to 543, and the number of beds nearly tripled from 37,849 to 106,265.[8]

The 1950 Mental Hygiene Law financially incentivized families to seek treatment for their mentally ill relatives at psychiatric facilities. For the first time, families could use services offered in public and private hospitals and clinics at little to no cost. The 1950 Law required that the government cover 95 percent of medical bills for outpatient psychiatric care such as consultations, medication, and daycare services. Some municipalities even covered the 5 percent copay, making psychiatric treatment essentially free for families. At the same time, the 1950 Law infringed upon patients' rights by allowing their legal guardians, usually a spouse or parent, to admit them into psychiatric wards without their consent. Prefectural governors, too, could place those who posed a risk to themselves or others in protective medical custody without the consent of patients or their families. The increased availability and affordability of psychiatric hospitals also led to the warehousing of mentally ill patients, in which families often abandoned relatives in hospitals with no intent of returning for them and hospitals held patients indefinitely. In a white paper published in 1956, the Ministry of Health and Welfare referred to the hospitalization of mentally ill individuals as "detainment" or "internment" (*shūyō*), rather than "hospitalization" (*nyūin*), the term used for patients admitted to general hospitals.[9] Most assumed that patients in psychiatric hospitals would be treated more like prisoners than patients, with little intent to treat or ever release them.

In contrast to other places in the world where anti-psychiatric movements in the late 1960s led to the gradual deinstitutionalization of psychiatric patients, Japan witnessed a steady increase in hospitalization in the four decades after the passage of the 1950 Mental Hygiene Law.[10] From 1961 to 1999, the number of hospitals and beds tripled.[11] Along with increased financial support from the state for both hospitals and families, the development of first-generation antipsychotics lowered the cost of maintaining psychiatric hospitals by reducing the number of nurses and orderlies employed. The demographic shift to cities and the growth of nuclear families, which reduced the availability of physical space and family members to care for those with mental illness, further increased demand for psychiatric facilities. Criticism of the often-low-quality inpatient care at psychiatric facilities certainly appeared over the decades and efforts to create more community mental health programs persisted, but for the most part, individuals were hospitalized at an unprecedented rate, making institutionalization the norm for patients with chronic and severe mental illnesses.[12]

Yet the crucial role of the family did not disappear. As this book has shown, family and other institutions existed as nodes in a broad network of care. Although outpatient services became more affordable from the 1950s, families still looked after the daily needs of the patient at home. Today, many patients attend daytime outpatient care and return to their families at the end of the day.[13] There has also been a shift to promoting "independent living," driven by the development of second-generation antipsychotic medication in the 1980s and 1990s, which enable even the severely mentally ill to live outside a psychiatric ward.[14] Even in cases of inpatient services, families have been compelled to care for their relatives within hospitals. Recruited as unpaid auxiliary caregivers, family members provide nonmedical services such as feeding the patient, cleaning the room, and doing the patient's laundry.[15]

Unsurprisingly, the family members tasked with providing such in-hospital care are usually women. Despite the increased availability and affordability of hospital-based care from the 1950s onward, the centrality of family and women's caregiving labor has not faded.[16]

Women's Labor and the Postwar Home as "Caregiving Center"

Women became the normative caregivers in the home at the turn of the twentieth century. In the preceding Edo period, women and men had both performed reproductive and productive labor in the home. But in the late nineteenth century, increasing numbers of middle- and upper-class urban households experienced a gendered division of labor that designated the daily tasks of caregiving as women's work. The Civil Code of 1898 legalized the inferior status of women within families, too, helping to devalue the work they performed to sustain the well-being of their kin. Nearly all observers, critics, and even women themselves took women's caregiving labor for granted. What appeared as the work and responsibility of "family" in legal codes, documents, and paperwork were, in fact, usually those of women in everyday life.

In the post–World War II period, the burden of familial responsibility for the mentally ill or otherwise ailing fell perhaps even more intensely on the shoulders of women than ever before. Although the revised Civil Code of 1948 abolished the legal status of the household (*ie*) and absolute authority of the male household head, conservative politicians and bureaucrats averse to promoting government-sponsored social welfare fought to retain the clause about family obligation. The "duty of support" for indigent and otherwise needy members continued to fall to parents, children, siblings, and "relatives living together."[17] At the same time, the Japanese economy grew in the 1950s and 1960s, resulting in husbands securing jobs that paid well enough so that women could stay at home without paid employment. One of the most conspicuous changes in urban middle- and upper-class family life was the disappearance of men from the home.[18] Not all women stayed at home, of course, but as in the early twentieth century, the status of "housewife" became an aspiration for married women, including those who engaged in wage labor.[19] Government and companies, too, came to see the housewife as integral to the postwar drive for economic growth, so much so that corporations created programs to train housewives in rationalizing and modernizing domestic work that would create more efficient and less stressful home environments, which would in turn allow men to dedicate themselves to their work outside

the home.[20] In this way, the postwar period witnessed a shift from the patriarchal household to a family system centered on the woman as household
manager and mother.[21]

The home thus became "a kind of caregiving center in postwar society,"
a place where women created a "warm, supportive, nurturant atmosphere
for husbands and children."[22] As wives and mothers, women tended to the
bodily health and needs of their families, essentially sustaining Japanese
social welfare through an idealized and feminized care characterized as
"warm, supportive, nurturant," even though the demands of such care were
constant and often exhausting. Even if actual daily care did not meet such
ideals, or female caregivers suffered intensely as a result, the expectation
that "the family"—a palatable term with culturally essentialist associations
that obscured the disproportionate burden placed on women's labor—
provide the physical and emotional care necessary to sustain "public
regimes of productivity" became a hallmark of the second half of the twentieth century.[23]

Such expectations of feminized caregiving extended beyond the home, as
seen in the case of *tsukisoi*, or female aides in psychiatric and general hospitals
who acted as one-on-one companions and servants for a male or female patient. The term *tsukisoi* is composed of two characters, the first derived from
the same verb "to attach" (*tsuku*) as in "fox attachment" (*kitsune tsuki*) and the
second meaning "nearness" or "aid." Since the nineteenth century when general hospitals were first built, families had been tasked to choose a member
or acquaintance to stay in the hospital with a patient as their bedside companion and caretaker. In the following decades, families began hiring *tsukisoi*
as substitute caretakers.[24] As a study of *tsukisoi* in three small psychiatric
hospitals in the late 1950s shows, *tsukisoi* were middle-aged "sub-professional
nurses" who had little to no training and were often in constant attendance
to a patient, especially when the latter was undergoing treatment.[25] The
tsukisoi served meals, washed garments, and talked with the patient, all the
while sleeping besides him or her in a separate cot. During times of treatment
when a patient might be heavily sedated for two weeks, the *tsukisoi* spoon-
fed the patient, sponged their bodies, cleaned urine and feces, and touched
and soothed during periods of anxiety. Once recovered from the treatment,
patients were guided by *tsukisoi* in order to relearn basic skills of walking,
eating, toileting, and bathing. The physical and emotional intimacy between
patient and *tsukisoi* has been characterized as "motherly," suggesting that the
psychiatric hospital was a site to which the domestic ideals of motherly behavior and care had been extended.[26]

Yet *tsukisoi* and others who performed "motherly" roles in postwar Japanese society might be seen in another way. The example of *tsukisoi* suggests that families, patients, and hired caretakers were involved in the creation of the feeling of family through processes of providing and receiving care. Such feelings were embodied and expressed in acts of caregiving that at times turned to neglect and abandonment in ways that suggest the extent to which "family" was contingent upon care. The family as a social unit or the role of a motherly caretaker, in other words, was neither automatic nor natural, as this book has shown. They were instantiated through acts of gendered labor to varying degrees. People affected by the Japanese child-welfare system—the children growing up in state care, adoptive or foster parents, and bureaucrats in charge of child welfare placements—are especially aware of the ways in which kinship ties are contingent and emerge over time, rather than being fixed to genetics and descent.[27] In the same way that such contingencies are obvious to children and caretakers who do not belong to normative family forms, the domestic management of madness uncovers the contradictions and exploitations involved in sustaining "family," both on paper and in lived everyday life.

The valuation of "family" in the decades after World War II, especially the assumed presence of the stay-at-home mother and wife, has sustained what one psychiatrist has recently called "Japanese-style treatment" (Nihonryū no chiryō) for mental illness: "private coping, and subsidized and socially legitimate spaces for rest, but not necessarily cure—a kind of warehousing of the nonfunctional in hopes that, over time, they will eventually rehabilitate and rejoin society."[28] Anthropologist Amy Borovoy has suggested that the persistence of this kind of private coping and custody exposes how Japanese society is generally "anti-psychiatric," which does not entail an explicit opposition to psychiatry, but rather a tendency to avoid labeling and diagnosing individuals in ways that will permanently distinguish them from their peers. There exists, Borovoy explains, "a web of ideas and institutions that militate against pathologizing the individual and that, instead, make it possible to view a vast array of human differences and distress as potentially manageable and containable through reliance on self-discipline, coping and support from family and others."[29] As a result, those who cannot accommodate the demands of "normal" life are usually offered custodial forms of care, which women in families are expected to provide. The expectation of the attentive care and sheer endurance of wives, mothers, and daughters (or at times hired female help) continues to reinforce the idea that mental, emotional, and even social distress is tractable and manageable through the "right" kind of familial socialization, even as the female providers of such care, as proud of their sacrifice and endurance as they sometimes may be, become sick themselves.

The Work of Gendering Madness

The notion that experiences of madness were differentiated by gender persisted into the postwar era. This book has traced the ways in which gendered notions of madness performed various kinds of cultural work during times of rapid social and economic changes. Diagnoses such as hysteria, neurasthenia, and menstrual psychosis earlier in the century helped people make sense of shifting gender norms and roles as Japan experienced rapid urbanization, imperial expansion, and capitalist growth. Many medical, criminological, legal, and government commentators invoked hysteria as a reactionary response to changes in women's roles in the spheres of political activism, higher education, and paid employment. Hysteria stabilized meanings of binary gender difference, especially as they intersected with those of age, class, and ability. It naturalized, in other words, the division between masculine and feminine forms of mental, emotional, and physical distress. Women diagnosed with these gendered ailments often implicitly rejected them, turning instead to the realm of kin and family to make sense of their illnesses. But they, too, engaged with the diagnoses, if only to make them intelligible in the contexts of their lives and in their own terms.

Various gendered understandings of madness went in and out of fashion over the course of the twentieth century. Some, like neurasthenia, faded almost completely from medical and popular discourse. In its place, *noirōze*, or "neurosis," became the 1950s catchword for allegedly pathological conditions caused by rapid social and economic changes, many of which were related to gender roles and the family, in the postwar period.[30] A popular slogan of 1955 was "the age of neurosis" (*noirōze jidai*), a phrase created in the wake of several well-publicized suicides that year.[31] Other diagnoses, like "path of blood" (*chi no michi*), which patent medicine advertisers and other popular medical writers in the 1890s and 1900s had pronounced as the indigenous form of "hysteria," lived on in various parts of the country. One ethnographic study of a rural village in northern Honshu in the 1980s suggested that middle-aged women regularly invoke *chi no michi* to discuss physical ailments at the end of menstruation, including dizziness, palpitations, headaches, and stiff shoulders.[32] A later study in areas as varied as Kobe City and a forestry village in Shiga prefecture showed that nearly all the interviewed women had at least a vague sense of what the term meant, but those living in remote regions spoke about it with more specificity. "*Chi no michi* is a kind of hysteria, I think," one woman said, "with headaches, and irritability. In fact, I told my friends I might have it when I had a bad spell a few years ago."[33] Like hysteria, *chi no michi* continues to function as a polysemic term, with many possible meanings existing at once. Some interviewed women thought *chi no michi* was a mostly psychological condition, whereas others saw it as bodily and physical. Most agreed that it was connected in one way or another to the female reproductive cycle, with difficult childbirth foretelling challenges at the end of one's reproductive years, for example.

Even as the names of diagnoses changed, the idea that women's reproductive functions caused mental, emotional, and physical distress stubbornly persisted across the twentieth century and beyond. Consider discussions of a medical diagnosis known as "nonspecific complaints" (*futei shūso*), often referred to as "medically unexplained symptoms" elsewhere in the world.[34] More commonly associated with women than men in Japan, "nonspecific complaints" encompass symptoms like headaches, coldness (*hieshō*), shoulder stiffness (*kata kori*), dizziness, nervousness, premenstrual pain, depression, and more. In 1980, three doctors working in a large Tokyo hospital wrote a book for the general public in which they claimed that such symptoms resulted from "chronic infectious pelvic disease" (*mansei kotsubannai kansenshō*).[35] They wrote that damage to the fallopian tubes, uterus, and vagina during miscarriages, abortions, childbirth, and menstruation could lead to bacterial infection, which could then affect the autonomic nervous system. A related diagnosis known as "autonomic nervous system disorder" (*jiritsu shinkei shicchōshō*) became popularized in the 1970s and 1980s as a catch-all diagnosis for nonspecific symptomatology, usually in women.[36] Some physicians have explained the higher incidence of "autonomic nervous system disorder" in women by pointing to, again, female reproductive systems, claiming that hormonal changes before and after menstruation and menopause affect the autonomic nervous system. Others fall back on essentialist notions of women as being more innately prone to nervousness than men.

Women respond to catch-all diagnoses like "autonomic nervous system disorder" in various ways. Many feel relieved when diagnosed with what sounds like a scientific and medically valid condition because it serves to legitimate and substantiate their pain. In the face of their families who usually do not recognize the reality and validity of their female relatives' suffering, the diagnosis confers validation while shielding the women from having to grapple directly with emotionally and socially difficult interpersonal issues. But some women do not necessarily seek or accept a medical diagnosis like "autonomic nervous system disorder." Like the women diagnosed with hysteria or menstrual psychosis in the 1920s and 1930s, women in the past few decades have continued to explain their pain in the family vernacular, a language that situates their bodily and psychic pain in the context of their intimate relationships of kin and community. They attribute physical symptoms associated with autonomic nervous disorders like allergies, asthma, and stiff shoulders to troubles in their family life. When interviewed in the 1980s, one woman in her mid-fifties described how her headaches and bouts of dizziness were mostly certainly attributable to a poorly functioning autonomic nervous system, but the latter was the result of "a bodily imbalance" resulting from difficult changes in her family life, such as her daughter leaving for middle school and therefore not needing her mother's help as much and the woman's husband experiencing stress at work. Another woman in her early fifties complained about similar symptoms and, without ever consulting a doctor declared, "I've got autonomic nervous disorder. It's a psychological thing (*seishinteki*). I have to work with my husband every day in business, and sometimes it causes problems."[37] Women readily invoke a widely known and accepted diagnosis, but sometimes just as entry points. Their symptoms are rendered intelligible only once they interpret them within the context of their intimate and domestic lives.

The tendency to interpret one's bodily and psychic health through the framework of kinship reinforces—or perhaps is the result of—the lack of a public narrative about the structural reasons for women's mental distress. This is not the case for men. As anthropologist Junko Kitanaka has shown, men have recourse to a widely accepted narrative that their depression is caused by chronic and excessive "overwork" (*karō*), which is commonly expected of employees in many Japanese companies. Since the 2000s, many victims and their families have successfully sued companies for pushing employees to suicide and depression, expecting them to work punishingly long hours even as a prolonged economic recession has led to diminishing job security. Although women have been among the plaintiffs, mental distress caused by "overwork" is usually associated with men. In contrast to male narratives of work-induced depression, those of women do not invoke social and economic injustices as plausible causes of illness. Nor are their narratives as uniform and socially legible as those of men. The concept of "overwork" in Japan is masculinized and does not extend into the feminized home or similar domestic settings. Domestic work, in other words, is not legible as "work." For physicians and family members, women's distress usually lacks "the clear shape of work-induced depression that a burned-out salaryman would be able to present, for instance, simply by stating his hours of overwork."[38]

Women's descriptions of their pain instead reflect how they are compelled to assume an array of roles with competing demands, with stress and fatigue deriving from usually both the workplace and the home. One fifty-nine-year-old woman, for instance, spoke of various sources of domestic and work-related stress when asked what she thought was the cause of her depression. In recent years she had been mediating a major conflict among her the staff at the daycare she directed while trying to manage issues at home, including a bankruptcy in the extended family and her son getting married and moving away, all without the help of a supportive husband. "I was so exhausted every day that I couldn't shake off the feeling of tiredness at the end of the day," she said.[39] These narratives of interlinked domestic, emotional, and professional issues are often taken less seriously than those of men by doctors and family members. Psychiatrists recognize the multiple and complex sources of stress for women, but at the same time tend to see women as suffering from psychologically-induced depression (neurotic depression), while treating men for biological depression (endogenous depression). The latter has always been more highly regarded in twentieth-century Japanese psychiatry.[40]

When women, whether in the early twentieth century or now, invoke aspects of their professional, domestic, and emotional lives and labors to explain their distresses, they are theorizing the structural features of the gender system in which they are embedded. Some scholars have suggested that women in Japan do not see the connection between social structures and female subordination, protesting their stress simply "by griping and gossiping about their immediate family members" or taking medication.[41] But "griping and gossiping" can be political acts. Women engage and experiment with feminized diagnoses like hysteria, menstrual psychosis, "path of blood," and autonomic nervous system disorder as a means of creating a theoretical framework for themselves that resonates with the realities of their lives. In their interactions with psychiatrists, relatives, and friends, they parse plausible causes of their bodily, psychic, and emotional pain. Women's general mistrust of doctors in Japan means that they usually do not indiscriminately accept medical opinions. Women may not have public narratives available to them that discuss their pain as a product of structural inequities, but their turn to the domain of kinship should not be dismissed as a lack of awareness about structural issues. Nor should it be seen as a relegation of their distress to the supposedly lowly realm of the domestic. Indeed, their invocation of kinship and domesticity resists the usual consignment of the domestic to a lower status. It gestures instead to the broader gender inequities through which the domestic realm is positioned as inferior.

The gendered understandings of the causes and care of madness produced within domestic settings at the turn of the twentieth century laid the groundwork for the designation of the family in the post–World War II period until today as a "natural" locus of care for those suffering from mental afflictions. Women and families have continually navigated changes in laws, political regimes, public health policies, economic development, and cultural crises to forge workable structures and cultures of care for those considered mad. The state and its supporters compelled women and families to follow a litany of directives and regulations since the late nineteenth century but offered little to no financial and social assistance with everyday care. Despite the spread of state-funded inpatient and outpatient psychiatric care since the 1950s, those with mental and conditions varying degrees of severity—from schizophrenia and depression to social withdrawal and autonomic nervous system disorder—are compelled to rely on their kin networks to serve as the primary managers of their care.

In recent decades, grassroots social movements have mobilized women and others to demand the redistribution of the responsibilities and costs of care among family, community, market, and state. Activists have called for an expansion of what has been called "social care," which entails the creation of a care infrastructure consisting of public and private, formal and informal sectors to help alleviate inequities among caregivers and receivers.[42] Yet the expansion of public care provision in the past three decades, even as it relieves some of the care burdens of women in families, has not necessarily translated to more gender-equitable social welfare thinking and policy making. Policies continue to rely on unpaid caretaking by women, and the notion that women ought to be responsible for family well-being strongly persists.[43] As seen in cases of doctors and family members dismissing and essentializing women's complaints and pain as effects of their personalities and gendered bodies, normative ideas and relations of gender have not changed enough for "social care" to serve as more than a policy response offering a limited solution to just one part of a deeply entrenched gender system. In other words, despite some successes in the redistribution of care provision, the gender system itself persists.

Family and kinship often reinforce the normative gender system, but they can also serve as ways to question it and theorize experiences that counter it. This is possible as long as definitions of "family" remain capacious, embracing the various modes through which kinship ties can be made and unmade. This book's focus on family-based management of madness in turn-of-the-twentieth century Japan has illuminated women's caregiving labor, supernatural foxes, and female sociality as examples of such modes of filiation that occurred alongside and in tension with more conventional legal and biological ones. Close attention to the sites of encounters in which such claims to kinship were made has enabled a deeper analysis of women's experiences of the gender system—how they creatively worked within and against it in order to generate vernacular languages that, above all, made sense to them in their everyday lives. Both back then and now, women's domestic labor, caregiving, and illness are crucial not only in the realm of managing mental illness, but those of elderly care, childrearing, and household welfare as well. Attuning to the longer histories and specificities of women's experiences within each context is one way of ensuring that much that lies outside normative structures and cultures of family and care can become visible.

Notes

INTRODUCTION

1. Case 1 in Shimamura Shun'ichi, "Shimane kenka kohyōbyō torishirabe hōkoku," *Tōkyō igakkai zasshi* 6, no. 6 (1892): 1–18; 7, no. 3 (1893): 24–39. Reprinted in *Kindai shomin seikatsushi*, ed. Minami Hiroshi et al. (Tokyo: San'ichi shobō, 1984–1988), 20: 44–72; Nakamura Kokyō, *Hisuterii no ryōhō* (Tokyo: Shufu no tomosha, 1932), 195–198; Akihito Suzuki, "Between Two Psychiatric Regimes: Migration and Psychiatry in Early Twentieth-Century Japan," in *Migration, Ethnicity, and Mental Health: International Perspectives, 1840–2010*, ed. Angela McCarthy and Catharine Coleborne (New York and London: Routledge, 2012), 150–151.

2. Akihito Suzuki, "Therapy, Care, and Punishment: The Family and the Psychiatric Hospital in Tokyo c. 1920–1945." Paper presented at The Seminar in the Department of History at Johns Hopkins University, October 31, 2016; Akihito Suzuki, "Psychiatric Hospitals, Domestic Strategies and Gender Issues in Tokyo c. 1920–1945," *History of Psychiatry* 33, no. 3 (forthcoming 2022).

3. Sheldon Garon, "State and Family in Modern Japan: A Historical Perspective," *Economy and Society* 39, no. 3 (2010): 317–336.

4. For recent works on the global rise of (colonial) psychiatry and other sciences of mind, see Emily Baum, *The Invention of Madness: State, Society, and the Beijing Insane, 1900–1937* (Chicago: University of Chicago Press, 2018); Emily Baum and Howard Chiang, eds., "Histories and Cultures of Mental Health in Modern East Asia: New Directions," *History of the Behavioral Sciences* 57, no. 3 (Summer 2021): 239–242; Debjani Das, *House of Madness: Insanity and Asylums of Bengal in Nineteenth-Century India* (New Delhi: Oxford University Press, 2015); Claire Edington, *Beyond the Asylum: Mental Illness in French Colonial Vietnam* (Ithaca, NY: Cornell University Press, 2019); Omnia El Shakry, *The Arabic Freud: Psychoanalysis and Islam in Modern Egypt* (Princeton, NJ: Princeton University Press, 2017); Jennifer Lambe, *Madhouse: Psychiatry and Politics in Cuban History* (Chapel Hill: University of North Carolina Press, 2017); Kah Seng Loh, "Mental Illness in Singapore: A History of a Colony, Port City, and Coolie Town," *East Asian Science, Technology and Society* 10, no. 2 (2016): 121–140;

Manuella Meyer, *Reasoning against Madness: Psychiatry and the State in Rio de Janeiro, 1830–1944* (Rochester, NY: University of Rochester Press, 2017); Harry Yi-Jui Wu and Wen-Ji Wang, eds., "Making and Mapping Psy Sciences in East and Southeast Asia," *East Asian Science, Technology and Society* 10, no. 2 (June 2016): 109–120; Nan Osei Quarshie, "Contracted Intimacies: Psychiatric Nursing Conspiracies in the Gold Coast," *Politique africaine* 157 (2020): 91–110.

5. Edward Shorter, *A History of Psychiatry: From the Era of the Asylum to the Age of Prozac* (New York: John Wiley & Sons, 1997), 34.

6. Megan Vaughan and Sloan Mahone, eds., *Psychiatry and Empire* (Basingstoke and New York: Palgrave Macmillan, 2007); Janice Matsumura, "Eugenics, Environment, and Acclimatizing to Manchukuo: Psychiatric Studies of Japanese Colonies," *Nihon ishigaku zasshi* 56, no. 3 (2010): 329–350; Theodore Jun Yoo, *It's Madness: The Politics of Mental Health in Colonial Korea* (Berkeley: University of California Press, 2016).

7. *Seishinbyō* was the literal translation of the German medical term *Geisteskrankheit*, or "sickness of spirit," which is often translated into English as "mental disease" or "mental illness." In early Japanese psychiatric textbooks, *seishinbyō* was the common translation for the German word *Psychose*, or psychosis, too. Here I use "madness" as well as "mental affliction" as generic terms for mental and emotional conditions considered abnormal, strange, or otherwise inexplicable in their historical contexts; "psychosis" as a specialist term used among psychiatrists; and "mental illness" as a term developed in medical and psychiatric discourse in the late nineteenth century that became integrated into a vernacular lexicon to describe psychosomatic abnormalities.

8. On the creation of Meiji biomedical systems and public health, see William Johnston, *The Modern Epidemic: A History of Tuberculosis in Japan* (Cambridge, MA: Council on East Asian Studies, Harvard University, 1995), 167–184; Susan Burns, "Constructing the National Body: Public Health and the Nation in Nineteenth-Century Japan," in *Nation Work: Asian Elites and National Identities*, ed. Timothy Brook and Andre Schmid (Ann Arbor: University of Michigan Press, 2000): 17–28; Ruth Rogaski, *Hygienic Modernity: Meanings of Health and Disease in Treaty-Port China* (Berkeley: University of California Press, 2004), 136–164; Kasahara Hidehiko and Kojima Kazutaka, *Meiji ki iryō eisei gyōsei no kenkyū* (Kyoto: Mineruva Shobō, 2011); Hōgetsu Rie, Kindai *nihon ni okeru eisei no tenkai to juyō* (Tokyo: Tōshindō, 2010). On the Meiji state's regulation of medicinal markets and pharmaceuticals, see Timothy Yang, *A Medicated Empire: The Pharmaceutical Industry and Modern Japan* (Ithaca, NY: Cornell University Press, 2021), 19–37.

9. Hoi-eun Kim, *Doctors of Empire: Medical and Cultural Encounters between Imperial Germany and Meiji Japan* (Toronto: University of Toronto Press, 2014).

10. For an overview of the spread of psychiatry in the Japanese empire, see Kazamatsuri Hajime, *Kindai seishin igakushi kenkyū: Tōkyō daigaku gasshūkoku gaichi no seishin igaku* (Tokyo: Chūōkōron jigyō shuppan, 2012).

11. Susan Burns, "Contemplating Places: The Hospital as Modern Experience in Meiji Japan," in *New Directions in the Study of Meiji Japan,* ed. Helen Hardacre and Adam L. Kern (Leiden: Brill, 1997), 702–718; Omata Wa'ichirō, *Seishinbyōin no kigen: kindai hen* (Tokyo: Ōta Shuppan, 2000); Okada Yasuo, *Shisetsu Matsuzawa byōinshi: 1879–1980* (Tokyo: Iwasaki Gakujutsu Shuppansha, 1981); Kanekawa Hideo, *Seishinbyōin no shakaishi* (Tokyo: Seikyūsha, 2009).

12. Hyōdō Akiko, *Seishinbyō no nihon kindai: tsuku shinshin kara yamu shinshin e* (Tokyo: Seikyūsha, 2008).

13. Satō Masahiro, *Seishin shikkan gensetsu no rekishi shakaigaku: "kokoro no yamai" wa naze ryūkyōsuru no ka* (Tokyo: Shin'yōsha, 2013).

14. Janice Matsumura, "State Propaganda and Mental Disorders: The Issue of Psychiatric Casualties among Japanese Soldiers during the Asia-Pacific War," *Bulletin of the History of Medicine* 78, no. 4 (Winter 2004): 804–835; Janice Matsumura, "Eugenics, Environment, and Acclimatizing to Manchukuo" ; Eri Nakamura, "Psychiatrists as Gatekeepers of War Expenditure: Diagnosis and Distribution of Military Pensions in Japan during the Asia-Pacific War," *East Asian Science, Technology and Society* 13, no. 1 (2019): 57–75; Serizawa Kazuya, *"Hō" kara kaihōsareru kenryoku: hanzai, kyōki, hinkon, soshite Taishō demokurashii* (Tokyo: Shinyōsha, 2001); Oda Susumu, ed., *"Hentai shinri" to Nakamura Kokyō: Taishō bunka e no shinshikaku* (Tokyo: Fuji Shuppan, 2001).

15. Akihito Suzuki, "The State, Family, and the Insane in Japan, 1900–45," in *The Confinement of the Insane: International Perspectives, 1800–1965,* ed. Roy Porter and David Wright (Cambridge: Cambridge University Press, 2003), 193–225. Original statistics in Kure Shūzō and Kashida Gorō, *Seishin byōsha shitaku kanchi no jitsujyō oyobi sono tōkeiteki kansatsu* (Tokyo: Sōzō shuppan, 2000 [1918]).

16. Elizabeth Lunbeck, *The Psychiatric Persuasion: Knowledge, Gender, and Power in Modern America* (Princeton, NJ: Princeton University Press, 1994). Also see Eva Illouz, *Saving the Modern Soul: Therapy, Emotions, and the Culture of Self-Help* (Berkeley: University of California Press, 2008).

17. Kure Shūzō and Kashida Gorō, *Seishin byōsha shitaku kanchi no jitsujyō oyobi sono tōkeiteki kansatsu* (Tokyo: Sōzō shuppan, 2000 [1918]).

18. Hashimoto Akira, ed., *Chiryō no basho to seishin iryōshi* (Tokyo: Nihon Hyōronsha, 2010); Christopher Harding, Iwata Fumiaki, and Yoshinaga Shin'ichi, eds., *Religion and Psychotherapy in Modern Japan* (Abingdon and New York: Routledge, 2015).

19. Another example is Shichiyama Byōin on the outskirts of Osaka. See Honda Yoshiharu, Suzuki Hideo, Honda Hideharu, and Irisawa Satoshi, "Chihō toshi seishinbyōin ni okeru sagyōryōhō no kusawake," *Seishin shinkeigaku zasshi* 111, no. 9 (2009): 1047–1054.

20. Susan Burns, "Reinvented Places: 'Tradition,' 'Family Care' and Psychiatric Institutions in Japan," *Social History of Medicine* 32 (February 2019): 99–120; Nakamura Osamu, *Rakuhoku Iwakura to seishinryō: seishinbyō kanja kazokuteki kango no dentō no keisei to shōshitsu* (Tokyo: Sekai shisōsha, 2013).

21. Hashimoto, ed., *Chiryō no basho*; Hashimoto Akira, *Seishin byōsha to shitaku kanchi* (Tokyo: Rikka Shuppan, 2011).

22. See Peter Bartlett and David Wright, eds., *Outside the Walls of the Asylum: The History of Care in the Community, 1750–2000* (New Brunswick, NJ: The Athlone Press, 1999); David Wright, "Getting Out of the Asylum: Understanding the Confinement of the Insane in the Nineteenth Century," *Social History of Medicine* 10 (1997): 137–155; Patricia Prestwich, "Family Strategies and Medical Power: 'Voluntary' Committal in a Parisian Asylum, 1876–1914," *Journal of Social History* 27 (1994): 799–818; Joseph Melling and Bill Forsythe, eds., *Insanity, Institutions and Society, 1800–1914: A Social History of Madness in Comparative Perspective* (London: Routledge, 1999); Akihito Suzuki, *Madness at Home: The Psychiatrist, the Patient, and the Family in England, 1820–1860* (Berkeley: University of California Press, 2006); Edington, *Beyond the Asylum*; Baum, *The Invention of Madness*.

23. Edington, *Beyond the Asylum*, 6–8.

24. Baum, *The Invention of Madness*, 75.

25. W. Evan Young, "Domesticating Medicine: The Production of Familial Knowledge in Nineteenth-Century Japan," *Historia Scientiarum* 27, no. 2 (2018): 127–149. On home-based care in an earlier period, see Andrew Edmund Goble, "Women and Medicine in Late 16th Century Japan: The Example of the Honganji Religious Community in Osaka and Kyoto as Recorded in the Diary of Physician Yamashina Tokitsune," *Asia Pacific Perspectives* 14, no. 1 (2016): 51–52.

26. On Edo-period poor relief, see Maren Ehlers, *Give and Take: Poverty and the Status Order in Early Modern Japan* (Cambridge, MA: Harvard University Asia Center, 2018).

27. Garon, "State and Family," 320.

28. On translations and interpretations of *ie*, see Kathleen Uno, "Questioning Patrilineality: On Western Studies of the Japanese *Ie*," *Positions* 4 (Winter 1996): 569–594.

29. On laws and policies concerning the establishment of the new family registration system (*koseki*) in the early Meiji period, see Fukushima Masao, "Meiji yonen kosei hō no shiteki zentei to sono kōzō," in *Kosei seido to "ie" seido*, ed. Fukushima Masao (Tokyo: Tokyo Daigaku Shuppankai, 1959): 94–169; Ninomiya Shūhei, "Kindai koseki seido no kakuritsu to kazoku no tōsei," in *Koseki to mibun tōroku*, ed. Toshitani Nobuyoshi, Kamata Hiroshi, and Hiramatsu Hiroshi (Tokyo: Waseda Daigaku Shuppanbu, 2005): 146–164.

On the uses of family registration records in enforcing public health measures such as compulsory sterilizations, detentions, and quarantines, as well as in collecting data and statistics about disease outbreaks, see Yuki Terazawa, *Knowledge, Power, and Women's Reproductive Health in Japan, 1690–1945* (n.p.: Palgrave Macmillan, 2018), 129; Kobayashi Takehiro, *Kindai nihon to koshū eisei* (Tokyo: Yūzankaku, 2001): 1–12, 39–57; Ozaki Kōji, "1879-nen korera to chihō eisei seisaku no tankan: Aichi-ken wo jirei to shite," *Nihonshi kenkyū* 418 (June 1997): 41–48.

30. There is extensive scholarship on the *ie* and "*ie* system" as a legal institution and an ideology through which the Meiji state structured "the Japanese family" and the "family-state," which then influenced family formations and law in the Japanese empire in the first half of the twentieth century as well. Representative works include Kawashima Takeyoshi, *Ideorogii to shite no kazoku seido* (Tokyo: Iwanami Shoten, 1957); Ito Mikiharu, *Kazoku kokkakan no jinruigaku* (Kyoto: Mineruva Shobō, 1982); Ueno Chizuko, *Kindai kazoku no seiritsu to shūen* (Tokyo: Iwanami Shoten, 1994); Muta Kazue, *Senryaku to shite no kazoku: kindai Nihon no kokumin kokka keisei to josei* (Tokyo: Shinyōsha, 1996). For a more extensive list of foundational works on *ie* and family from the seventeenth century onward, see Mary Elizabeth Berry and Marcia Yonemoto, eds., *What Is a Family?: Answers from Early Modern Japan* (Berkeley: University of California Press, 2019): 261–266.

    Other normative models of family such as *katei* (usually translated as "home" or "family"), which competed and overlapped with ideas and practices related to *ie*, were created by participants of an emerging mass-market press. See Muta Kazue, "Images of the Family in Meiji Periodicals: The Paradox Underlying the Emergence of the 'Home,'" trans. Marcella S. Gregory, U.S.-Japan Women's Journal, English Supplement 7 (1994): 53–71; Nishikawa Yūko, "The Changing Form of Dwellings and the Establishment of the Katei (Home) in Modern Japan," trans. Manko Muro Yokokawa, U.S.-Japan Women's Journal, English Supplement 8 (1995): 3–36; Jordan Sand, *House and Home in Modern Japan: Architecture, Domestic Space, and Bourgeois Culture, 1880–1930* (Cambridge, MA: Harvard University Asia Center, 2003); Kathryn Ragsdale, "Marriage, the Newspaper Business, and the Nation-State: Ideology in the Late Meiji Serialized *Katei Shōsetsu*," *Journal of Japanese Studies* 24, no. 2 (Summer 1998): 229–255.

    On the extension, reformulation, and adaptation of Japanese laws and ideologies of family and kinship in the Japanese empire, see, e.g., Sungyun Lim, *Rules of the House: Family Law and Domestic Disputes in Colonial Korea* (Berkeley: University of Calfironia Press, 2019); Chen Chao-ju, "*Sim-pua* under the Colonial Gaze: Gender, 'Old Customs,' and the Law in Taiwan under Japanese Imperialism," in *Gender and Law in the Japanese Imperium*, ed. Susan L. Burns and Barbara J. Brooks (Honolulu: University of Hawai'i Press, 2013): 189–218; Barbara J. Brooks, "Japanese Colonialism, Gender, and Household Registration: Legal Reconstruction of Boundaries," in *Gender and Law in the Japanese Imperium*, ed. Susan L. Burns and Barbara J. Brooks (Honolulu: University of Hawai'i Press, 2013): 219–239; Tadashi Ishikawa, "Human Trafficking and Intra-Imperial Knowledge: Adopted Daughters, Households, and Law in Imperial Japan and Colonial Taiwan, 1919–1935," *Journal of Women's History* 29, no. 3 (2017): 37–60.

31. Some historians have argued that sick-nursing in the Edo period was primarily the responsibility of men, but persuasive arguments against such an interpretation exist. See W. Evan Young, "Family Matters: Managing Illness in Late Tokugawa Japan, 1750–1868" (PhD diss., Princeton University, 2015), 40–46.

32. Kathleen Uno, "Women and Changes in the Household Division of Labor," in *Recreating Japanese Women, 1600–1945*, ed. Gail Lee Bernstein (Berkeley: University of California Press, 1991), 25.

33. Uno, "Women and Changes in the Household Division of Labor," 36.

34. On "good wife, wise mother," see Koyama Shizuko, *Ryōsai kenbo to iu kihan* (Tokyo: Keisō Shobō, 1991); Kathleen Uno, "Womanhood, War, and Empire: Transmutations of 'Good Wife, Wise Mother' before 1931," in *Gendering Modern Japanese* History, ed. Barbara Molony and Kathleen Uno (Cambridge, MA: Harvard University Asia Center, 2005), 493–519; Mark Jones, *Children as Treasures: Childhood and the Middle Class in Early Twentieth Century Japan* (Cambridge, MA: Harvard University Asia Center, 2010), 116–170.

35. Miyake Akimasa, "Female Workers of the Urban Lower Class," in *Technology Change and Female Labour in Japan*, ed. Nakamura Masanori (Tokyo: United Nations Press, 1994), 97–131; Kathleen Uno, "One Day at a Time: Work and Domestic Activities of Urban Lower-Class Women in Early Twentieth-Century Japan," in *Japanese Women Working*, ed. Janet Hunter (London and New York: Routledge, 1993), 37–68; Margit Nagy, "Middle-Class Working Women during the Interwar Years," in *Recreating Japanese Women, 1600–1945*, ed. Gail Lee Bernstein (Berkeley: University of California Press, 1991), 199–216.

36. Elyssa Faison, *Managing Women: Disciplining Labor in Modern Japan* (Berkeley: University of California Press, 2007), 8–10; Robert J. Smith, "Making Village Women into 'Good Wives and Wise Mothers' in Prewar Japan," *Journal of Family History* 8, no. 1 (1983): 70–84.

37. Mary Fissell, "Women, Health, and Healing in Early Modern Europe," *Bulletin of the History of Medicine* 82, no. 1 (2008): 13; Kathleen Brown, *Foul Bodies: Cleanliness in Early America* (New Haven, CT: Yale University Press, 2011).

38. See, e.g., Patricia Tsurumi, *Factory Girls: Women in the Thread Mills of Meiji Japan* (Princeton, NJ: Princeton University Press, 1990); Janet Hunter, *Women and the Labour Market in Japan's Industrialising Economy: The Textile Industry before the Pacific War* (London: RoutledgeCurzon, 2003); Faison, *Managing Women*; Sachiko Sone, "Japanese Coal Mining: Women Discovered," in *Women Miners in Developing Countries: Pit Women and Others*, ed. Kuntala Lahiri-Dutt and Martha Macintyre (Aldershot, England, and Burlington, VT: Ashgate, 2006), 51–72; Susan Newell, "Women Primary School Teachers and the State in Interwar Japan," in *Society and the State in Interwar Japan*, ed. Elise K. Tipton (London and New York: Routledge, 1997), 17–41; Miriam Silverberg, *Erotic Grotesque Nonsense: The Mass Culture of Japanese Modern Times* (Berkeley: University of California Press, 2006), 73–107; Elise K. Tipton, "Pink Collar Work: The Café Waitress in Early Twentieth Century Japan," *Intersections: Gender, History and Culture in the Asian Context* 7 (March 2002), http://intersections.anu.edu.au/issue7/tipton.html; Alisa Freedman, Laura Miller, and Christine R. Yano, eds., *Modern Girls on the Go: Gender, Mobility, and Labor in Japan* (Palo Alto, CA: Stanford University Press, 2013).

39. Yamashita Mai, *Kangofu no rekishi: yorisou senmonshoku no tanjō* (Tokyo: Yoshikawa Kōbunkan, 2017); Aya Takahashi, *The Development of the Japanese Nursing Profession: Adopting and Adapting Western Influences* (London and New York: RoutledgeCurzon, 2004); Aya Homei, "Birth Attendants in Meiji Japan: The Rise of the Biomedical Birth Model and a New Division of Labour," *Social History of Medicine* 19, no. 3(2006): 407–424; Homei Aya, "'Seijō san' to 'Kindai eisei': Kindai sanba no senmon bunya wo meguru poritikkusu," *Seibutsugaku shi kenkyū*, no. 70 (December, 2002): 1–16; Julie Rousseau, *Enduring Labors: The "New Midwife" and the Modern Culture of Childbearing in Early Twentieth Century Japan* (PhD diss., Columbia University, 1998), 69-113; Terazawa, *Knowledge, Power, and Women's Reproductive Health in Japan*, 125-176. On similar women's work in the Japanese empire, see Sonja M. Kim, *Imperatives of Care: Women and Medicine in Colonial Korea* (Honolulu: University of Hawai'i Press, 2019).

40. One important exception is Kathleen S. Uno, *Passages to Modernity: Motherhood, Childhood, and Social Reform in Early Twentieth-Century Japan* (Honolulu: University of Hawai'i Press, 1999).

41. Shimizu Michiko, *"Jochū" imēji no katei bunkashi* (Tokyo: Sekai Shisōsha, 2004); Ōkuda Akiko, "Jochū no rekishi," in *Onna to otoko no jikū—Nihon joseishi saikō*, ed. Ōkuda Akiko (Tokyo: Fujiwara Shoten, 1995), 5:376–410; Kōnosuke Odaka, "Redundancy Utilized: The Economics of Female Domestic Servants in Pre-war Japan," in *Japanese Women Working*, ed. Janet Hunter (London: Routledge, 1993), 16–36; Miri Nakamura, "The Cult of Happiness: Maid, Housewife, and Affective Labor in Higuchi Ichiyō's 'Warekara,'" *Journal of Japanese Studies* 41, no. 1 (Winter 2015): 45–78; Jiyoung Suh, "The Gaze on the Threshold: Korean Housemaids of Japanese Families in Colonial Korea," *positions* 27, no. 3 (2019): 437-468.

42. For analyses of the relationship between women's paid employment and unpaid domestic work, see Yoshiko Miyake, "Doubling Expectations: Motherhood and Women's Factory Work under State Management in Japan in the 1930s and 1940s," in *Recreating Japanese Women, 1600–1945*, ed. Gail Lee Bernstein (Berkeley: University of California Press, 1991), 267–295; Kathleen Uno, "One Day at a Time: Work and Domestic Activities of Urban Lower-Class Women in Early Twentieth-Century Japan," in *Japanese Women Working*, ed. Janet Hunter (London: Routledge, 1993), 37–68.

43. Arthur Kleinman, "Caregiving: The Divided Meaning of Being Human and the Divided Self of the Caregiver," in *Rethinking the Human*, ed. J. Michelle Molina and Donald K. Swearer with Susan Lloyd McGarry (Cambridge, MA: Center for the Study of World Religions, Harvard Divinity School: 2010), 18. Care has long been treated by philosophers, sociologists, and anthropologists as a crucial site of ethics, a place where the moral dynamics of everyday life unfold and develop in a relationship between a caregiver and a recipient. On feminist care ethics, see, e.g., Sandra Laugier, "The Ethics of Care as a Politics of the Ordinary," New Literary History 46, no. 2 (2015): 217–240; Ueno Chizuko, *Kea no shakaigaku: tojisha shuken no fukushishakai e* (Tokyo: Ōta shuppan, 2011).

44. Lisa Stevenson, *Life beside Itself: Imagining Care in the Canadian Arctic* (Berkeley: University of California Press, 2014), 3.

45. There is a rich debate among anthropologists about how to re-conceptualize "care" in ways that foreground its ambiguities, tensions, and surprises. See, e.g., Stevenson, *Life beside Itself;* Angela Garcia, *The Pastoral Clinic: Addiction and Dispossession along the Rio Grande* (Berkeley: University of California Press, 2010); Felicity Aulino, *Rituals of Care: Karmic Politics in an Aging Thailand* (Ithaca, NY: Cornell University Press, 2019); Clara Han, *Seeing Like a Child: Inheriting the Korean War* (New York: Fordham University Press, 2021); Arthur Kleinman, *The Soul of Care: The Moral Education of a Husband and Doctor* (New York: Viking, 2019); Jocelyn Lim Chua, *In Pursuit of the Good Life: Aspiration and Suicide in Globalizing South India* (Berkeley: University of California Press, 2014).

46. Kure Shūzō and Kashida Gorō, *Seishin byōsha shitaku kanchi no jitsujyō oyobi sono tōkeiteki kansatsu* (Tokyo: Sōzō shuppan, 2000 [1918]).

47. Sara Pinto, *Daughters of Parvati: Women and Madness in Contemporary India* (Philadelphia: University of Pennsylvania Press, 2014), 3.

48. On the creation of non-biological kinship through acts of caregiving in contemporary Japan, see Kathryn E. Goldfarb, "'Coming to Look Alike': Materializing Affinity in Japanese Foster and Adoptive Care," *Social Analysis* 60, no. 2 (Summer 2016): 47–64, and "Beyond Blood Ties: Intimate Kinships in Japanese Foster and Adoptive Care," in *Intimate Japan: Ethnographies of Closeness and Conflict,* ed. Alison Alexy and Emma E. Cook (Honolulu: University of Hawai'i Press, 2018): 181–198.

49. For related studies on evolving notions of blood and kinship from the eighteenth century onward, see, e.g., Nishida Tomomi, *Chi no shisō: Edo Jidai no Shiseikan* (Tokyo: Kenseisha, 1995); Jennifer Robertson, "Hemato-Nationalism: The Past, Present, and Future of 'Japanese Blood,'" *Medical Anthropology: Cross-Cultural Studies in Health and Illness* 31, no. 2 (2012): 93–112.

50. In tracing intimate ties that were made and unmade through acts and denials of caregiving, this book draws on a wide range of works that have historicized the invention of "kinship" as a theory of biological relatedness by anthropologists and evolutionary scientists in the nineteenth century; illuminated the ways in which kinship is enacted, performed, or practiced around the world; and offered ways of loosening "kinship" from its biological and hereditary associations. See, e.g., Lisa Hofmann-Kuroda, "The Tree of Life: The Politics of Kinship in Meiji Japan (1870–1915) (PhD diss., University of California Berkeley 2018); Ken Ito, *An Age of Melodrama: Family, Gender, and Social Hierarchy in the Turn-of-the-Century Japanese Novel* (Stanford, CA: Stanford University Press, 2008); Joseph M. Pierce, *Argentine Intimacies: Queer Kinship in an Age of Splendor, 1890–1910* (Albany, NY: State University of New York Press, 2019); Jessica Marie Johnson, *Wicked Flesh: Black Women, Intimacy, and Freedom in the Atlantic World* (Philadelphia: University of Pennsylvania Press, 2020); Brigitte Fielder, *Relative*

Races: Genealogies of Interracial Kinship in Nineteenth-Century America (Durham, NC: Duke University Press, 2020); Judith Butler, *Antigone's Claims: Kinship between Life and Death* (New York: Columbia University Press, 2000).

51. Akihito Suzuki, "Were Asylums Men's Places? Male Excess in the Asylum Population in Japan in the Early Twentieth Century," in *Psychiatric Cultures Compared: Psychiatry and Mental Health Care in the Twentieth Century*, ed. Gijswijit-Hofstra et al. (Amsterdam University Press, 2005), 295–311.

52. European medical theories, too, had long constructed the category of feminine hysteria in opposition to that of a masculine nervous disorder whose name shifted over the centuries, at times referred to as "melancholy" and at others as "hypochondria" and "neurasthenia." See Elaine Showalter, "Hysteria, Feminism, and Gender," in *Hysteria beyond Freud*, ed. Sander Gilman et al. (Berkeley: University of California Press, 1993), 292; Elaine Showalter, *The Female Malady: Women, Madness, and Culture in England, 1830–1980* (New York: Pantheon Books, 1985).

53. Mental illness was often differentiated by both gender and class. Whereas middle- and upper-class men were frequently diagnosed with neurasthenia, working-class men suffered from "traumatic neurosis" (*gaishosei shinkeishō*) as a result of workplace accidents. At the same time, "traumatic neurosis" spanned class divides, as seen in widespread diagnoses among Japanese soldiers before 1945. See Satō, *Seishin shikkan gensetsu no rekishi shakaigaku*, 273–317; Matsumura, "State Propaganda and Mental Disorders."

54. See, e.g., the entry for hysteria in the first authoritative Japanese psychiatry textbook. Kure Shūzō, *Seishinbyōgaku shūyō* (Tokyo, 1895), 259–71. For more on translations and interpretations of hysteria among early Japanese psychiatrists, see Chapter 3, notes 47 and 50.

55. Carroll Smith-Rosenberg and Charles Rosenberg, "The Female Animal: Medical and Biological Views of Woman and Her Role in Nineteenth-Century America," *Journal of American History* 60, no. 2 (1973): 335.

56. The pathologization of women's emotions and reproductive functions occurred across societies in the turn-of-the-twentieth-century world, but the political, social, and cultural conditions in which it gained (and sometimes lost) traction varied. Hysteria in the United States, for instance, was racialized as an affliction of "over-civilized" white women, whereas in Japan the preeminent "disease of civilization" was male neurasthenia. Women in the Japanese empire, whether colonized or not, affluent or impoverished, were said to contract the "less-civilized" illness of hysteria. See Laura Briggs, "The Race of Hysteria: 'Overcivilization' and the 'Savage' Woman in Late Nineteenth-Century Obstetrics and Gynecology," *American Quarterly* 52, no. 2 (2000): 246–273; Marta Hanson, "Depleted Men, Emotional Women: Gender and Medicine in the Ming Dynasty," *NAN NÜ* 7, no. 2 (Leiden: Brill, 2005), 288; and Mark Driscoll, "Empire in Hysterics," in *Absolute Erotic, Absolute Grotesque: The Living, Dead, and Undead in Japan's Imperialism, 1895–1945* (Durham, NC: Duke University Press, 2010), 81–100. On

global discourses of women's mental pathologies, see also Frank Dikötter, *Sex, Culture, and Modernity in China: Medical Science and the Construction of Sexual Identities in the Early Republican Period* (Hong Kong: Hong Kong University Press, 1995); Hugh Shapiro, "Pathologizing Marriage: Neuropsychiatry and the Escape of Women in Early Twentieth-Century China," in *Psychiatry and Chinese History*, ed. Howard Chiang (London: Pickering and Chatto, 2014), 129–141; Cassia Roth, *A Miscarriage of Justice: Women's Reproductive Lives and the Law in Early Twentieth-Century Brazil* (Stanford, CA: Stanford University Press, 2020); Ornella Moscucci, *The Science of Woman: Gynaecology and Gender in England, 1800–1929* (Cambridge: Cambridge University Press, 1990); Emily Martin, *The Woman in the Body: A Cultural Analysis of Reproduction* (Boston: Beacon Press, 1987); Caroline Bledsoe, *Contingent Lives: Fertility, Time, and Aging in West Africa* (Chicago: University of Chicago Press, 2002); Hilary Marland, *Dangerous Motherhood: Insanity and Childbirth in Victorian Britain* (New York: Palgrave Macmillan, 2004); Julie Parle, *States of Mind: Searching for Mental Health in Natal and Zululand, 1868–1918* (Scottsville, South Africa: University of KwaZulu-Natal Press, 2007), 128–164; Vincenza Mazzeo, "The Discursive Origins of 'Bantu Gynecology' in the *South African Medical Journal*, 1910–1940" (MA Thesis, Carleton University); Kristin Ruggiero, *Modernity in the Flesh: Medicine, Law, and Society in Turn-of-the-Century Argentina* (Stanford, CA: Stanford University Press, 2004); Sander Gilman, "Black Bodies, White Bodies: Toward an Iconography of Female Sexuality in Late Nineteenth-Century Art, Medicine, and Literature," *Critical Inquiry* 12, no. 1 (1985): 204–242.

57. On sexology, see Sabine Frühstück, *Colonizing Sex: Sexology and Social Control in Modern Japan* (Berkeley: University of California Press, 2003).

58. See, e.g., Moscucci, *The Science of Woman*, 102; and Martin, *The Woman in the Body*.

59. On comparative East Asian contexts, see Charlotte Furth, *A Flourishing Yin: Gender in China's Medical History, 960–1665* (Berkeley: University of California Press, 1999); Hsiu-fen Chen, "Between Passion and Repression: Medical Views of Demon Dreams, Demonic Fetuses, and Female Sexual Madness in Late Imperial China," *Late Imperial China* 32, no. 1 (June 2011): 51–82. Yi-Li Wu's work illuminates how highly educated male physicians promoted the idea "that women's illnesses were essentially no different from men's" as a way of distinguishing themselves from non-scholarly amateur doctors and midwives who assumed that women's reproductive capacity made their bodies fundamentally different from men's. See Yi-Li Wu, *Reproducing Women: Medicine, Metaphor, and Childbirth in Late Imperial China* (Berkeley: University of California Press, 2010).

60. Keiko Daidoji, "What a Household with Sick Persons Should Know: Expressions of Body and Illness in a Medical Text of Early Nineteenth-Century Japan" (PhD diss., University of London, 2009), 197. Classical Chinese medical texts, too, often stressed the "specific agency of emotion" in cases of female illnesses. See Furth, *A Flourishing Yin*, 87–88.

61. Satoko Shimazaki, *Edo Kabuki in Transition: From the Worlds of the Samurai to the Vengeful Female Ghost* (New York: Columbia University Press, 2016), 150–193.

62. Arthur Kleinman, *The Illness Narratives: Suffering, Healing, and the Human Condition* (New York: Basic Books, 1988), 122.

63. Veena Das and Renu Addlakha, "Disability and Domestic Citizenship: Voice, Gender, and the Making of the Subject," *Public Culture* 13, no. 3 (2001): 520.

64. See, e.g., Shigehisa Kuriyama, "The Historical Origins of *Katakori*," *Japan Review* 9 (1997): 127–149.

65. Veena Das, *Affliction: Health, Disease, Poverty* (New York: Fordham University Press, 2015), 2–3.

66. Sandra Laugier, "The Ethics of Care as a Politics of the Ordinary," *New Literary History* 46, no. 2 (Spring 2015): 217–240.

67. On the use of the term "time-knots" to evoke such notions of disjointed and layered temporalities, see Dipesh Chakrabarty, *Provincializing Europe: Postcolonial Thought and Historical Difference* (Princeton, NJ: Princeton University Press, 2000), 112.

CHAPTER 1

1. *Yomiuri shinbun*, March 10, 1882, 2.

2. Fox attachment in the post-1868 era has mostly been studied under the rubric of the "anti-superstition campaign." See Kawamura Kunimitsu, *Genshi suru kindai kūkan: meishin, byōki, zashikirō, aruiwa rekishi no kioku* (Tokyo: Seikyūsha, 1990); Kawamura Kunimitsu, *Hyōi no kindai to poritikusu* (Tokyo: Seikyūsha, 2007); Gerald Figal, *Civilization and Monsters: Spirits of Modernity in Meiji Japan* (Durham, NC: Duke University Press, 1999); Jason Ananda Josephson, *The Invention of Religion in Japan* (Chicago: University of Chicago Press, 2012); Michael Dylan Foster, *Pandemonium and Parade: Japanese Monsters and the Culture of Yōkai* (Berkeley: University of California Press, 2009).

3. *Yomiuri shinbun*, September 11, 1932, 9.

4. James Fujitani, "The Jesuit Hospital in the Religious Context of Sixteenth-Century Japan," *Japanese Journal of Religious Studies* 46, no. 1 (2019): 93; Andrew Edmund Goble, "Women and Medicine in Late 16th Century Japan: The Example of the Honganji Religious Community in Osaka and Kyoto as Recorded in the Diary of Physician Yamashina Tokitsune," *Asia Pacific Perspectives* 14, no. 1 (2016): 51–52.

5. For a related discourse on *ki* and aesthetic eccentricity in the Edo period, see W. Puck Brecher, *The Aesthetics of Strangeness: Eccentricity and Madness in Early Modern Japan* (Honolulu: University of Hawai'i Press, 2013).

6. Junko Kitanaka, *Depression in Japan: Psychiatric Cures for a Society in Distress* (Princeton, NJ: Princeton University Press), 26.

7. Itahara Kazuko and Kuwabara Haruo, "Edo jidai koki ni okeru seishin shōgai no shogu (3)," *Shakai mondai kenkyū* 49, no. 2 (2000): 183–200; Hiruta Genshirō, *Hayariyamai to kitsunetsuki: kinsei shomin no iryō jijō* (Tokyo: Misuzu shobō, 1985).

8. Although *kanpō* physicians rarely specialized in "madness," many created classification systems for what they called *kan*, which has been translated as "mental disorders" that included disease categories that scholars have translated as "psychosis" (*kyō*), "fright disorder" (*kyō*), epilepsy (*ten*), and dementia (*chigai*). Still, they did not always distinguish between body and mind, seeing madness as a symptom with roots in the whole organism. See Hiruta Genshirō, "Japanese Psychiatry in the Edo Period (1600–1868)," *History of Psychiatry* 13 (2002): 131–151; Shigehisa Kuriyama, "The Historical Origins of *Katakori*," *Japan Review* 9 (1997): 127–149. Similar conceptions of madness can be found in classical Chinese medical thought. See Furth, *A Flourishing Yin*, 87–88.

9. Keiko Daidoji, "Treating Emotion-Related Disorders in Japanese Traditional Medicine: Language, Patients and Doctors," *Culture, Medicine, and Psychiatry* 37 (March 2013): 63.

10. Hiruta Genshirō, "Japanese Psychiatry in the Edo Period (1600–1868)."

11. Keiko Daidoji, "What a Household with Sick Persons Should Know," 184–189.

12. Ishizuka Takatoshi, *Nihon no tsukimono: zokushin wa ima mo ikite iru* (Tokyo: Miraisha, 1972); Yoshida Teigo, *Nihon no tsukimono: shakai jinruigakuteki kōsatsu* (Tokyo: Chūō Kōronsha, 1974); Carmen Blacker, *The Catalpa Bow: A Study of Shamanistic Practices in Japan* (London: George Allen & Unwin Ltd., 1975); Komatsu Kazuhiko, *Hyōrei shinkōron* (Tokyo: Hatsubaisho Gendai Jānarizumu Shuppankai, 1982).

13. Michael Dylan Foster, "Haunting Modernity: *Tanuki*, Trains, and Transformation in Japan," *Asian Ethnology* 71, no. 1 (2012): 9.

14. Hiruta, *Hayariyamai to kitsunetsuki*, 56–126.

15. Nakamura Teiri, *Kitsune no Nihon shi: Kinsei kindai hen* (Tokyo: Nihon Editā Sukūru Shuppanbu, 2003); Pamela D. Winfield, "Curing with *Kaji*: Healing and Esoteric Empowerment in Japan," *Japanese Journal of Religious Studies* 32, no. 1 (2005): 107–130.

16. Shinmura Taku, *Nihon bukkyō no iryōshi* (Tokyo: Hōsei Daigaku Shuppan Kyoku, 2013).

17. For instance, the Soto Zen temple of Kōganji popularized cults centered on Buddhist deities and bodhisattvas by selling and distributing talismans that were ingested or ritually cast into rivers as prayers for healing. See Duncan Williams, *The Other Side of Zen: A Social History of Sōtō Zen Buddhism in Tokugawa Japan* (Princeton, NJ: Princeton University Press, 2004), 86–116.

18. See, e.g., Daniel Trambaiolo, "Native and Foreign in Tokugawa Medicine," *The Journal of Japanese Studies* 39, no. 2 (2013): 299–324; Benjamin Elman, "Sinophiles and Sinophobes in Tokugawa Japan: Politics, Classicism, and Medicine during the Eighteenth Century," *East Asian Science, Technology and Society* 2, no. 1 (2008): 93–121; Ann Bowman Jannetta, *The Vaccinators: Smallpox, Medical Knowledge, and the 'Opening' of Japan* (Stanford, CA: Stanford University Press, 2007).

19. Susan L. Burns, "Nanayama Jundō at Work: A Village Doctor and Medical Knowledge in Nineteenth Century Japan," *East Asian Science, Technology, and Medicine* 29 (2008): 63.

20. Cited in Hiruta, "Japanese Psychiatry in the Edo Period," 137–138.

21. Kitamura Ryotaku, "Tohō ron [1817]," in *Iseidō sōsho*, ed. Kure Shūzō (1923; repr., Kyoto: Shinbunkaku, 1970), 46.

22. Nakamura Teiri, *Kitsune no Nihon shi*, 301–304.

23. W. Evan Young, "Domesticating Medicine: The Production of Familial Knowledge in Nineteenth-Century Japan," *Historia Scientiarum* 27, no. 2 (2018): 130.

24. Young, "Domesticating Medicine," 148.

25. See, e.g., Allan G. Grapard, "Japan's Ignored Cultural Revolution: The Separation of Shinto and Buddhist Divinities in Meiji ("Shimbutsu Bunri") and a Case Study: Tōnomine," *History of Religions* 23, no. 3 (1984): 240–265; James Ketelaar, *Of Heretics and Martyrs in Meiji Japan: Buddhism and Its Persecution* (Princeton: Princeton University Press, 1993); Trent E. Maxey, *The "Greatest Problem": Religion and State Formation in* Meiji Japan (Cambridge, MA: Harvard University Asia Center, 2014); and Sarah Thal, "Redefining the Gods: Politics and Survival in the Creation of Modern Kami," *Japanese Journal of Religious Studies* 29 (2002): 379–404.

26. Quoted in Jason Ananda Josephson, *The Invention of Religion in Japan* (Chicago: University of Chicago Press, 2012), 181.

27. Barbara Ambros, "Clerical Demographics in the Edo-Meiji Transition: Shingon and Tōzanha Shugendō in Western Sagami," *Monumenta Nipponica* 64 (2009): 118.

28. On the coinage of the term "superstition" in Meiji Japan, see Josephson, *The Invention of Religion in Japan*, 177.

29. Cited in Kawamura Kunimitsu, *Genshi suru kindai kūkan: meishin, byōki, zashikirō, aruiwa rekishi no kioku* (Tokyo: Seikyūsha, 2006), 61–62.

30. *Yomiuri shinbun*, November 10, 1875, 1.

31. *Chi no michi* was a widely evoked phrase for female health issues that triggered symptoms such as dizziness, palpitations, headaches, chilliness, stiff shoulders, and dry mouth. Beginning in the Edo period, the term evoked the circulation of blood throughout the body, as well as its stoppages and overflows. See Chapter 3: Hysteria in the Marketplace, as well as Satō Masahiro, *Seishin shikkan gensetsu no rekishi shakaigaku*, 190–199.

32. On similar newspaper accounts that censured religious healers in rural areas, see Ikegami Yoshimasa, "Local Newspaper Coverage of Folk Shamans in Aomori Prefecture," in *Folk Beliefs in Modern Japan*, ed. Inoue Nobutaka (Tokyo: Kokugakuin University, 1994), 9–91.

33. Barbara Ambros has shown that many Shingon clerics in the early 1870s in western Sagami, for instance, were originally agricultural cultivators who were "barely

able to sustain themselves with the fees of performing funerary services." Ambros, "Clerical Demographics in the Edo-Meiji Transition," 85.

34. Helen Hardacre, "Conflict between Shugendō and the New Religions of Bakumatsu Japan," *Japanese Journal of Religious Studies* 21, no. 2/3 (June–September 1994): 137–166.

35. Hoi-eun Kim, *Doctors of Empire*, 20–21; William D. Johnston, "Buddhism contra Cholera: How the Meiji State Recruited Religion Against Epidemic Disease," in *Science, Technology, and Medicine in the Modern Japanese Empire*, ed. David G. Wittner and Philip C. Brown (London: Routledge, 2016), 62–78; Akihito Suzuki and Mika Suzuki, "Cholera, Consumer and Citizenship: Modernisations of Medicine in Japan," in *The Development of Modern Medicine in Non-Western Countries*, ed. Hormoz Ebrahimnejad (London: Routledge 2008), 184–203; Susan Burns, "Bodies and Borders: Syphilis, Prostitution, and the Nation in Japan, 1860–1890," *U.S.-Japan Women's Journal*. English Supplement no. 15 (1998): 3–30.

36. Johnston, *The Modern Epidemic*, 174.

37. Although both Japanese and German terms contain words that are mostly commonly translated in English as "spirit," the terms referred to evolving notions of diseases of the mind, rather than supernatural beings or religious notions of the soul.

38. Hyōdō Akiko, *Seishinbyō no nihon kindai*, 40–64 and 93–115; Susan Burns, "Relocating Psychiatric Knowledge: Meiji Psychiatrists, Local Culture(s), and the Problem of Fox Possession," *Historia Scientiarum* 22, no. 2 (December 2012): 88–109.

39. Erwin Baelz, *Awakening Japan: The Diary of a German Doctor*, ed. Toku Baelz, trans. Eden and Cedar Paul (New York: Viking Press, 1932), 398. See also Hoi-eun Kim, *Doctors of Empire*.

40. On the medical journals in which Baelz's article was published, see Burns, "Relocating Psychiatric Knowledge," 97.

41. Erwin Baelz (Eruvin Berutsu), "Kohyō byōsetsu," *Iji shinbun*, no. 148 (1885): 21. On Baelz's ethnographic, anthropological, and medical work in Japan, see Yasui Hiroshi, *Berutsu no shōgai: kindai igaku dōnyū no chichi* (Kyoto: Shibunkaku, 1995); Wakabayashi Misako et al., eds., *Berutsu nihon bunka ronshū* (Tokyo: Tōkai daigaku shuppankai, 2001).

42. Shimamura Shun'ichi, "Shimane kenka kohyōbyō torishirabe hōkoku," *Tōkyō Igakkai Zasshi* 6, no. 6 (1892): 1–18; 7, no. 3 (1893): 24–39. Reprinted in *Kindai shomin seikatsushi*, ed. Minami Hiroshi et al. (Tokyo: San'ichi shobō, 1984–1988), 20:44–72. All citations of Shimamura's report below refer to the reprint. For a short biography of Shimamura, see Okada Yasuo, "Shimamura Shun'ichi shōden: hiun no seishinbyōgakusha," *Nihon ishigaku zasshi* 38, no. 4 (1992): 603–634; Araki Sōtarō, "Tokushimakenka no inugamitsuki oyobi tanukitsuki ni tsuite," *Chūgai iji shinpō* 485 (June 5, 1900): 5–12; Araki Sōtarō, "Tokushimakenka no inugamitsuki oyobi

tanukitsuki ni tsuite," *Chūgai iji shinpō* 486 (June 20, 1900): 15–29. Psychiatrist Morita Masatake conducted on-site observations in nearby Tosa. Morita Masatake, "Tosa ni okeru inugami ni tsuite," *Shinkeigaku zasshi* 3, no. 3 (1904): 129–130.

43. Shimamura, "Shimane kenka kohyōbyō torishirabe hōkoku," 45.

44. Araki, "Tokushima kenka no inugamitsuki," *Chūgai iji shinpō* 485, 5.

45. For instance, Kure Shūzō introduced the term "zōsōsho" (臓躁症) as the Japanese word for hysteria in the first major textbook of Japanese psychiatry, *Seishinbyōgaku shūyō* (1895). He likely adapted the term from the Chinese medical classic *Essential Medical Treasures of the Golden Chamber* (*Kinki yōryaku hōron*), which featured an ailment called *fujin zōsō* (婦人臓躁), or "women's mania." According to the classic, women who suffered from *zōsō* were either flooded with a sadness that made them cry or were possessed by spirits. Kure stripped the original Chinese term of the qualifier "*fujin*," or "women," briefly explaining that both women and men could be afflicted by *zōsō*, though he contended that young women between ages 20 and 30, as well as children, both boys and girls around age 10, were disproportionally affected by it. See Kure Shūzō, *Seishinbyōgaku shūyō* (Tokyo, 1895), 259–271; Ishii Atsushi, "Kamata Sekian Fujin zōsōsetsu kō," *Seishin igaku* 28, no. 5 (1986): 583–588.

46. Mark S. Micale, "On the 'Disappearance' of Hysteria: A Study in the Clinical Deconstruction of a Diagnosis," *Isis* 84, no. 3 (September 1993): 503. For a summary of late nineteenth-century medical understandings of hysteria, see Katrien Libbrecht, *Hysterical Psychosis: A Historical Survey* (New Brunswick, NJ: Transaction Publishers, 1995).

47. Richard von Krafft-Ebing, *Lehrbuch der Psychiatrie auf klinischer Grundlage für praktische Ärzte und Studierende*, 3rd ed. (Stuttgart: Verlag von Ferdinand Enke, 1888), 567. Here the translation is adapted from *Textbook of Insanity based on Clinical Observations for Practitioners and Students of Medicine*, trans. Charles Gilbert Chaddock (London: F. A. Davis Company, 1904), 493. In his first psychiatry textbook, Kure Shūzō drew heavily from Krafft-Ebing's work. Kure's description of hysteria closely resembles that of Krafft-Ebing. See Kure Shūzō, *Seishinbyōgaku shūyō* (Tokyo, 1895), 259–273.

48. Shimamura, "Shimane kenka kohyōbyō torishirabe hōkoku," 56.

49. Shimamura, "Shimane kenka kohyōbyō torishirabe hōkoku," 58.

50. Kadowaki Sakae, *Kōhyōbyō shinron* (1902; repr., Tokyo: Sōzō Shuppan, 2001).

51. Kure Shūzō, "Kōhyōbyō to 'hisuterii' to no kankei," *Katei eisei sōsho* 4 (1905): 63, 65, and 69.

52. Kure, *Seishinbyōgaku shūyō*, 1.

53. Hyōdō, *Seishinbyō no nihon kindai*, 111.

54. Blacker, *Catalpa Bow*, 51. Also see Ishizuka, *Nihon no tsukimono*.

55. Ishizuka, *Nihon no tsukimono*, 40. This origins story is recounted in Shimamura Shun'ichi, "Shimane kenka kohyōbyō torishirabe hōkoku," 51.

56. Foxes were also considered as agents of commercial prosperity in the worship of a Shinto divinity named Inari. By the end of the Edo period, Inari had become

one of the most ubiquitous and multifaceted objects of devotion in Japanese religious life, and Inari worship became the single most widely recognized focal point of fox imagery in Japan. See Karen Smyers, *The Fox and the Jewel: Shared and Private Meaning in Contemporary Japanese Inari Worship* (Honolulu: University of Hawai'i Press, 1999).

57. Thomas C. Smith, *The Agrarian Origins of Modern Japan* (Stanford, CA: Stanford University Press, 1959), 108–139; Conrad Totman, *Early Modern Japan* (Berkeley: University of California Press, 2005), 249.

58. Hayami Yasutaka, *Tsukimono-mochi meishin: sono rekishiteki kōsatsu* (Tokyo: Akashi shoten, 1999), 109–115.

59. Bathgate, *The Fox's Craft in Japanese Religion and Folklore*, 128.

60. Ann Waswo, "The Transformation of Rural Society, 1900–1950," in *The Cambridge History of Japan*, ed. John Whitney Hall et al. (Cambridge: Cambridge University Press, 1989), 6:544.

61. On agriculture and the local economy in Shimane prefecture, see Yukiko Kawahara, "Local Development in Japan: The Case of Shimane Prefecture from 1800–1930" (PhD diss., University of Arizona, 1990), 11–133.

62. For a thought-provoking historical comparison, see discussions of witchcraft in Europe, especially Robin Briggs, *Witches and Neighbors: The Social and Cultural Context of European Witchcraft* (New York: Penguin Books, 1998); Wolfgang Behringer, *Shaman of Oberstdorf: Chonrad Stoeckhlin and the Phantoms of the Night* (Charlottesville: University Press of Virginia, 1998); Stuart Clark, ed., *Languages of Witchcraft: Narrative, Ideology and Meaning in Early Modern Culture* (New York: St. Martin's Press, 2001); Stuart Clark, *Thinking with Demons: The Idea of Witchcraft in Early Modern Europe* (Oxford: Clarendon Press, 1997). For a synthesis of debates on the history of witchcraft, see Malcolm Gaskill, "The Pursuit of Reality: Recent Research into the History of Witchcraft," *Historical Journal* 51, no. 4 (2008): 1069–1088.

63. Shimamura, "Shimane kenka kohyōbyō torishirabe hōkoku," 55.

64. Araki, "Tokushima kenka no inugamitsuki," *Chūgai iji shinpō*, 486, 17.

65. Basil Hall Chamberlin, *Things Japanese: Being Notes on Various Subjects Connected with Japan for the Use of Travellers and Others* (London; Yokohama; Shanghai: John Murray; Kelly & Walsh, Ltd., 1905), 118.

66. Bathgate, *The Fox's Craft in Japanese Religion and Folklore*, 122.

67. The reference to the Siege of Osaka is most likely a reference to a series of battles in 1614 and 1615 in which the Tokugawa shogunate defeated the previously ruling Toyotomi clan. Shimamura, "Shimane kenka kohyōbyō torishirabe hōkoku," 65.

68. Envy arose from other reasons, too. When a thirty-five-year-old woman in the Ōhara district in Shimane prefecture showed signs of fox-spirit attachment, the "human-fox" (*ninko*) was said to have said the following: "I have come from the neighboring Yamamoto household. My household has five members. Your house only has two or three members. Yet even when sick, you work in the fields. You strive to accumulate money and get rich. You are truly greedy. I watch this from the

side, and there is no end to [my] feelings of jealousy, so I have come to attach myself to you." Shimamura, "Shimane kenka kohyōbyō torishirabe hōkoku," 56–57.

69. Araki, "Tokushima kenka no inugamitsuki," 15–16. Similarly, in sixteenth- and seventeenth-century Europe, neighbors routinely emphasized the malice and envy of the person accused of witchcraft. See Briggs, *Witches and Neighbors*, 166.

70. Shimamura, "Shimane kenka kohyōbyō torishirabe hōkoku," 64.

71. Shimamura, "Shimane kenka kohyōbyō torishirabe hōkoku," 45.

72. Shimamura, "Shimane kenka kohyōbyō torishirabe hōkoku," 44.

73. Akihito Suzuki and Mika Suzuki, "Cholera, Consumer, and Citizenship." For a rich analysis of popular consciousness and rumors during the early-Meiji cholera epidemics, see Sugiyama Hiroshi, "Bunmei kaikaki no hayariyamai to minshū ishiki: Meiji jūnendai no korera matsuri to korera sōdō," *Machida shiritsu jiyū minken shiryōkan* 2 (1988): 19–50.

74. See, e.g., Bettina Gramlich-Oka, "The Body Economic: Japan's Cholera Epidemic of 1858 in Popular Discourse," *East Asian Science, Technology, and Medicine* 30 (2009), 32–73; William Johnston, "Cholera and Popular Culture in Nineteenth Century Japan," *Historia Scientiarum* 27, no. 2: 174–198.

75. Takahashi Satoshi, *Bakumatsu orugi: korera ga yatte kita!* (Tokyo: Asahi shinbunsha, 2005), 63.

76. Takahashi, *Bakumatsu orugi*, 179–184; Duane B. Simmons, *Cholera Epidemics in Japan: With a Monograph on the Influence of the Habits and Customs of Races on the Prevalence of Cholera* (Shanghai: Statistical Department of the Inspectorate General of Customs, 1880), 5. Similarly imaginative spellings (*ateji*) for cholera included 虎列刺, 虎狼痢, and 虎狼理.

77. *Yomiuri shinbun*, February 5, 1880, 2.

78. Rokuhara Hiroko, "Local Officials and the Meiji Conscription Campaign," *Monumenta Nipponica* 60, no. 1 (2005): 83.

79. *Tōkyō nichinichi shinbun* 914, January 23, 1885. Reprinted in Okada Yasuo, *Nihon seishinka iryōshi* (Tokyo: Igaku Shoin, 2002), 116; and Nihon Ishi Gakkai, ed., *Zuroku Nihon iji bunka shiryō shūsei* (Tokyo: Sanichi Shobō, 1979), 180.

80. Okada Yasuo, *Nihon seishinka iryōshi* (Tokyo: Igaku Shoin, 2002), 116.

81. Cited in Hirota Masaki, *Sabetsu no shosō. Nihon kindai shisō taikei*, ed. Katō Shūichi (Tokyo: Iwanami Shoten, 1990), 22: 492.

CHAPTER 2

1. Cases 15 and 16 in Kure Shūzō, *Seishin byōsha shitaku kanchi no jikkyō* [hereafter *SBSK*] (Tokyo: Naimushō Eiseikyoku 1918), 19–22.

2. One important exception is Hashimoto Akira's foundational studies of home confinement, which examine how families inhabited spaces of confinement and responded to state and medical surveillance and intervention. See Hashimoto Akira, *Seishin byōsha to shitaku kanchi* (Tokyo: Rikka Shuppan,

2011); Hashimoto Akira, "Seishinbyōsha kangohōka no Okinawa (1900–1960) to shitakukanchi: Okinawaken kōbunshokan shozō shiryō no bunseki," *Shakai fukushi kenkyū* 22 (2020): 21–38. Studies of home confinement that focus on the role of families rarely analyze their everyday experiences living with confinement. See, e.g., Aoyama Yōji, "Seishinbyōsha no kazoku no yakuwari: seishinbyōsha kangōhō ni yoru kanri shisutemuu," *Kaihō shakaigaku kenkyū* 14 (2000): 116–133. Most studies have focused on the creation of the 1900 Custody Law, e.g., Akakura Takako, "Meiji 33 nen 'Seishinbyōsha kangohō' no mondaiten to shinhō seiritsu ni mukete no katsudō: Taishō 8 nen 'Seishinbyōinhō' seiritsu no haikei" [Kobe daigaku daigakuin hōgaku kenkyūkai hen], *Rokkōdai ronshū* 47, no. 3 (2001): 1–69; Nakatani Yōji, "Seishinbyōsha kangohō wa naze seitei saretaka," *Seishin igakushi kenkyū* 5, no. 1 (2001): 181–197; Nishikawa Kaoru, "Seishinbyōsha kangohō seitei ni kansuru ichikenkyū: seitei ito ni kansuru senkō kenkyū hihan," *Gendai shakai bunka kenkyū* 24 (2001): 143–160; Utsunomiya Minori, "Seishinbyōsha kangohō seiritsuzen no seishin shōgaisha taisaku," *Tōkai joshi daigaku kiyō* 26 (2006): 61–84; Okada Yasuo, *Nihon seishinka iryōshi* (Igaku shoin, 2002), 130–146.

3. Although domestic confinement of those considered mad was not unique to Japan, the extent of the legal obligations of care placed on families into the twentieth century was unusual. On families confining mentally troubled members in makeshift enclosures in the United States, Europe, Korea, China, and Indonesia, see James Moran, "Architectures of Madness: Informal and Formal Spaces of Treatment and Care in Nineteenth-Century New Jersey," in *Madness, Architecture, and the Built Environment: Psychiatric Spaces in Historical Context*, ed. Leslie Topp, James E. Moran, and Jonathan Andrews (New York: Routledge, 2007), 153–172; Edward Shorter, *A History of Psychiatry: From the Era of the Asylum to the Age of Prozac* (New York: John Wiley & Sons, 1997), 3–4; Zhiying Ma, "An Iron Cage of Civilization? Missionary Psychiatry, the Chinese Family and a Colonial Dialectic of Enlightenment," in *Psychiatry and Chinese History*, ed. Howard Chiang (London: Routledge, 2015), 91–110; Harry Minas and Hervita Diatri, "*Pasung*: Physical Restraint and Confinement of the Mentally Ill in the Community," *International Journal of Mental Health Systems* 2, no. 8 (2016), doi:10.1186/1752-4458-2-8; Fabien Simonis, "Mad Acts, Mad Speech, and Mad People in Late Imperial Chinese Law and Medicine," PhD diss., Princeton University, 2010; Theodore Jun Yoo, *It's Madness: The Politics of Mental Health in Colonial Korea* (Oakland: University of California Press, 2016), 139.

4. Statistical data on the number of mentally ill people in Japan, as well as the number of people who were confined at home or elsewhere, are notoriously unreliable for the late nineteenth century, but one government record suggests that in 1905 there were 29,931 individuals registered with local and prefectural offices as mentally ill patients, 4,400 of whom were confined either at home or in hospitals. In 1925, there were 54,673 registered patients, 4,814 of whom were confined at home and 2,411 in hospitals. By 1935, the number of registered patients had increased to 83,465, with 5,163 in hospitals and 7,188 confined at home. See *Isei hachijyūnen*

shi (Tokyo: Kōseishō imukyoku, 1955), 802–803. Cited in Hashimoto, *Shitaku kanchi*, 42–43.

5. Other common terms for confinement rooms included various spellings for *sashiko* (指子, 指籠, 差籠) and *uchiori* (内折). See Hiruta Genshirō, *Hayariyamai to kitsunetsuki: kinsei shomin no iryō jijō* (Tokyo: Misuzu shobō, 1985), 60. One of the earliest records of the term *zashikirō* can be found in an entry for "Zaxiqirô (ザシキロウ)" in a Japanese-Portuguese dictionary compiled by the Jesuits in 1603: "Sala, ou camara que se dá por irenico, ou estar preso em casa" ("Room, or chamber that pacifies, or to be caged at home." See *zashikirō* in Japan Knowledge Library, http://japanknowledge.com/library/.

6. Katsu Kokichi, *Musui dokugen: hoka* (Tokyo: Heibonsha, 1969 [1843]), 60. English translation available in Craig Teruko, trans., *Musui's Story: The Autobiography of a Tokugawa Samurai* (Tucson: University of Arizona Press, 1988), 68.

7. Katsu, *Musui dokugen*, 60.

8. Edo literature and poetry are laced with references to parlor prisons. One well-known example can be found in "Kibitsu no kama," a story from Ueda Akinari's *Ugetsu monogatari* (1776). For an analysis of confinement in Ueda's narrative, see Nakamura Masaichi, "*Ugetsu monogatari* Kibitsu no kama kō: Shōtarō to zashikirō," *Shōkei gakuin kenkyū kiyō* 4 (2010): 17–28. For a well-known literary representation of home confinement in the Meiji period, see Shimazaki Tōson, *Before the Dawn*, trans. William E. Naff (Honolulu: University of Hawai'i Press, 1987 [1929]).

9. Okada Hajime, ed., *Haifū yanagidaru zenshū*, 12 vols. (Tokyo: Sanseido: 1976–1978). For examples of *senryū* in English translation, see Makoto Ueda, trans., *Light Verse from the Floating World: An Anthology of Premodern Japanese Senryū* (New York: Columbia University Press, 1999).

10. *Haifū yanagidaru*, 1:281.

11. *Haifū yanagidaru*, 2:172.

12. *Haifū yanagidaru*, 12:140.

13. See Nakamura Masaichi, "*Ugetsu monogatari* Kibitsu no kama kō," 17–28.

14. *Haifū yanagidaru*, 2:212.

15. On the prison Denmachō, see Daniel Botsman, *Punishment and Power in the Making of Modern Japan* (Princeton, NJ: Princeton University Press, 2007).

16. *Haifū yanagidaru*, 1:79.

17. Itahara Kazuko and Kuwabara Haruo, "Edo jidai koki ni okeru seishin shōgai no shogu IV," *Shakai mondai kenkyū* 50 (2000): 79–94.

18. *Tame*-like places that existed in other cities such as Osaka, Nagasaki, and Kanazawa also probably admitted the mentally disturbed. See Itahara Kazuko and Kuwabara Haruo, "Edo jidai koki ni okeru seishin shōgai no shogu IV," *Shakai mondai kenkyū* 50 (2000): 80.

19. Hiruta, *Hayariyamai to kitsunetsuki*, 109–110.

20. Psychiatrist and historian Yamazaki Tasuku argued that Edo-period families were less inclined to confine relatives at home because of the family feuds that

such decisions might incite. See Yamazaki Tasuku, "Seishinbyōsha shogukō 4," *Shinkeigaku zashi* 34 (1932): 399–412.

21. Cited in Itahara and Kuwabara, "Edo jidai koki ni okeru seishin shōgai no shogu II," 106.

22. Itahara and Kuwabara, "Edo jidai koki ni okeru seishin shōgai no shogu II," 95. See also Hiruta, *Hayariyamai to kitsunetsuki.*

23. Katō Takashi, "Governing Edo," in *Edo and Paris: Urban Life and the State in the Early Modern Era*, ed. James L. MacClain, John M. Merriman, and Kaoru Ugawa (Ithaca, NY: Cornell University Press, 1997), 55.

24. See Carl Steenstrup, *A History of Law in Japan until 1868* (Leiden: E. J. Brill, 1991), 131; Hayami Akira, "The Myth of Primogeniture and Impartible Inheritance in Tokugawa Japan," *Journal of Family History* 8 (1983): 3–28; Aoi Okada and Satomi Kurosu, "Succession and the Death of the Household Head in Early Modern Japan: A Case Study of a Northeastern Village, 1720–1870," *Continuity and Change* 13 (1998): 143–166; Yamanaka Einosuke, "Merchant 'House' (Iye) and Its Succession in Kyoto during the Tokugawa Era," *Osaka University Law Review* 11 (1963): 47–58; and Saito Osamu, "Marriage, Family Labour and the Stem Family Household: Traditional Japan in a Comparative Perspective," *Continuity and Change* 15 (2000): 17–45.

25. See *Kyūbakufu hikitsugisho* (1868) vol. 14, the official records of the South-North City Magistrate of the city of Edo. Cited in Itahara Kazuko and Kuwabara Haruo, "Edo jidai koki ni okeru seishin shōgai no shogu II," *Shakai mondai kenkyū* 49 (2000). On succession customs of various status groups, including shopkeepers, merchants, and artisans, see Katakura Hisako, "Edo machikata ni okeru sōzoku," in *Sōzoku to kasan*, ed. Nagahara Kazuo and Yoshie Akiko (Tokyo: Yoshikawa Kōbunkan, 2003), 89–112.

26. Ishi'i Ryōsuke contends that the terms of confinement were strict for the mentally ill because they could unintentionally cause fires. See Ishi'i Ryōsuke, *Nihon sōzokuhō shi* (Tokyo: Sōbunsha, 1980), 80–83.

27. Cited in Umemori Naoyuki, "Modernization through Colonial Mediations: The Establishment of the Police and Prison System in Meiji Japan" (PhD diss., University of Chicago, 2002), 30–31.

28. *Keishichō futatsu ki dai 172 go.* Cited in Okada Yasuo, *Nihon seishinka iryōshi*, 130. See also Shiomitsu Takashi, "Seishin shōgaisha no Kazoku seisaku ni kan suru ikkōsatsu: hogosha seidō no hensen wo tegakari ni," *Fukushi kyōiku kaihatsu sentaa kiyō* 13 (2017), https://archives.bukkyo-u.ac.jp/rp-contents/FC/0014/FC00140L 073.pdf.

29. For examples of prefectural ordinances, see Okada Yasuo, Hashimoto Akira, and Komine Kazushige, eds., *Seishin shōgaisha mondai shiryō shūse* (Tokyo: Rikka shuppan, 2010–2011), 1:43–98.

30. Cited in Hashimoto, *Shitaku kanchi*, 22–25.

31. *Hōrei zensho* (Tokyo: Naikaku kanpōkyō, 1912), 87–92, https://dl.ndl.go.jp/info:ndljp/pid/788016/54.

32. The remaining thirteen articles explain the fines and punishments for wrongful confinement, that is, confinement without the approval of local authorities or with falsified documents. Submitting a falsified report could land a custodian in jail for up to one year. Doctors who falsified diagnosis forms were subject to similar penalties. Scholars have suggested that Diet members were motivated to include such articles in the Custody Law in the wake of the Soma Incident of 1884, a case of wrongful confinement of a former daimyo. See Hashimoto, *Seishinbyōsha to shitaku kanchi*, 20–21; Burns, "Constructing the National Body," 42; Utsunomiya Minori, "Seishinbyōsha kango hōan teishutsu ni itaru yōin ni kansuru kenkyū," *Shakaijigyōshi kenkyū* 36 (2009): 109–122; Nishikawa Kaoru, "Soma jiken to seishinbyōsha kangōhō seitei no kanren: senkō kenkyū rebū," *Gendai shakai bunka kenkyū* (Niigata daigaku daigakuin gendai shakai bunka kenkyūka) 26 (2003): 35–51.

33. Garon, "State and Family in Modern Japan," 320.

34. Wilhelm Röhl, ed., *History of Law in Japan since 1868* (Leiden: Brill, 2005), 168.

35. See Turan Kayaoğlu, *Legal Imperialism: Sovereignty and Extraterritoriality in Japan, the Ottoman Empire and China* (2010), 82–83; Michael R. Auslin, *Negotiating with Imperialism: The Unequal Treaties and the Culture of Japanese Diplomacy* (2006).

36. Hozumi Yatsuka, "Minpō idete, chūkō horobu," in *Meiji shisō shū* 2, vol. 31 of *Kindai Nihon shisō taikei*, ed. Matsumoto Sannosuke (Tokyo: Chikuma Shobō, 1977), 17. Originally published in *Hōgaku shinpō*, August 1891.

37. Garon, "State and Family in Modern Japan," 321.

38. Records of debates in the National Diet concerning the creation of the Custody Law, as well as all other related bills, laws, and ordinances, are available through the National Diet Library Japanese Laws database, https://hourei.ndl.go.jp/simple/detail?lawId=0000005995&current=-1.

39. "Seishinbyōsha kangōhō seitei no ken" (1899 September), reprinted in *Seishinshōgaisha mondai shiryō shūsei* 4 (Tokyo: Rikka shuppan), document 117, p. 4. See also Utsunomiya Minori, "Seishinbyōsha kangohō no 'kango' gainen no kenshō," *Shakai fukushi gaku* 51, no. 3 (2010): 68.

40. "Minpō," *Hōrei zensho* (1898). Translation of the Civil Code available in Ludwig Lönholm, *The Civil Code of Japan* (Tokyo: Kokubunsha, 1898).

41. Cited in Nishikawa Kaoru, "Seishinbyōsha kangohō seitei ni kansuru ichikenkyū," 151.

42. In practice, a range of family members became legal custodians. Among 235 legal custodians in the Kure report, 25% were birth fathers, 19.5% wives, 13.6% birth mothers, 8.9% older brothers, and 5.5% younger brothers. Others (less than 5% each) included grandfathers, adopted fathers, adopted mothers, older sisters, younger sisters, cousins, nieces, and nephews. *SBSK*, 107–108.

43. Ken Ito, *An Age of Melodrama*, 21–22.

44. Kitamura Harumatsu, *Seishinbyōsha kangohōrei jimon jitō roku* (Osaka: Keisatsubu, 1904). Reprinted in *Seishin shōgaisha mondai shiryō shūse*, ed. Okada Yasuo, Hashimoto Akira, and Komine Kazushige (Tokyo: Rikka shuppan, 2010–2011), 4:6–22.

45. On changes in prefectural laws after the passage of the national Custody Law, see Hashimoto, *Seishinbyōsha to shitaku kanchi*, 29–34.

46. Akihito Suzuki, "The State, Family, and the Insane in Japan, 1900–45," in *The Confinement of the Insane: International Perspectives, 1800–1965*, ed. Roy Porter and David Wright (Cambridge: Cambridge University Press, 2003), 193–225.

47. Kure Shūzō and Kashida Gorō, "Seishinbyōsha shitaku kanchi no jikkyō oyobi sono tōkeiteki kansatsu," *Tōkyō igakukai zasshi* 32, no. 10–13 (1918): 521–715. Most of the original reports of the team of psychiatrists are no longer available, with the exception of Saitō Tamao's surveys conducted in Gunma and Yamanashi prefectures in 1910 and 1911, respectively. See Saitō Tamao, "Gunma-ken kanka seishinbyōsha shitaku kanchi jyōkyō shisatsu hōkoku," in *Seishin shōgaisha mondai shiryō shūse*, ed. Okada Yasuo, Hashimoto Akira, and Komine Kazushige (Tokyo: Rikka shuppan, 2010–2011 [1910]), 4:43–65, and "Yamanashi kenka seishinbyōsha shitaku kanchi jyōkyō shisatsu hōkoku," in *Seishin shōgaisha mondai shiryō shūse*, ed. Okada Yasuo, Hashimoto Akira, and Komine Kazushige (Tokyo: Rikka shuppan, 2010–2011 [1911]), 4:66–90.

48. On the visual strategies used in the Kure report, see Yumi Kim, "Seeing Cages: Home Confinement in Early Twentieth-Century Japan," *Journal of Asian Studies* 77, no. 3 (2018): 635–658.

49. Hashimoto Akira, *Seishinbyōsha to shitaku kanchi*, 73–76; 213–215.

50. Case 21, *SBSK*, 25–26.

51. Gail Bernstein, "Women in the Silk-reeling Industry in Nineteenth Century Japan," in *Japan and the World: Essays on Japanese History and Politics in Honour of Ishida Takeshi*, ed., Gail Lee Bernstein and Haruhiro Fukui (London: Palgrave Macmillan, 1988), 55.

52. Case 37, *SBSK*, 36–37.

53. Case 83, *SBSK*, 68.

54. Case 82, *SBSK*, 67.

55. Case 85, *SBSK*, 69–70.

56. Case 59, *SBSK*, 52–53.

57. Criticism of the family as a site of caregiving for those considered mentally ill was not limited to Japan at the turn of the twentieth century. For a counterpoint to Kure's sympathy for the plight of impoverished Japanese families struggling to manage madness, see Zhiying Ma's work on American missionary doctors and psychiatrists, who condemned "the Chinese family" as a source of barbaric cruelty and abusive treatment and called for the hospitalization of those considered mad in newly-built asylums. See Zhiying Ma, "An Iron Cage of Civilization?"

58. *SBSK*, 129.

59. *SBSK*, 128.

60. Pinto, *Daughters of Parvati*, 11.

61. *SBSK*, 109–110. Other forms of violence, whether actual or potential, that led to confinement included murder, property damage, arson, theft, suicide threats, vagrancy, breaking into government offices (*kanga chinnyū*), and acts or words of disloyalty toward the emperor or imperial family.

62. Kure's report counted sixty-seven instances in which families confined relatives for "wandering outside, especially heading to remote places or the mountains." See *SBSK*, 109–110.

63. Cases 15 and 16, *SBSK*, 19–22.

64. Kure's report documented other locations for confinement rooms, such as in separate hut-like sheds in the yard (10.9%), as attachments to the main house (10.3%), inside clay-walled storehouses (6.9%), as stand-alone structures separate from the main house (4.6%), on the earthen floor in the work space of the house (4%), in makeshift edifices connected to storehouses (2.3%), in the kitchen (1.7%), or other places (2.9%). See *SBSK,* 113–114.

65. Residents of Tokyo and Osaka were usually hospitalized in a public or private hospital, but other prefectures did not have appropriate medical facilities, so individuals were confined in a rented room or in spaces dedicated to the mentally ill within quarantine facilities, relief centers (救護所 *kyūgojo*), and sanitaria (療養所 *ryōyōjo*). See *SBSK*, 132–133.

66. Case 99, *SBSK*, 78–79; "Kōro seishinbyōsha hōkoku" (Gunma ken: Takazaki shichō, 1906), in *Seishin shōgaisha mondai shiryō shūse*, ed. Okada Yasuo, Hashimoto Akira, and Komine Kazushige (Tokyo: Rikka shuppan, 2010–2011), 4:23–35.

67. Case 98, *SBSK*, 78.

68. Case 102, *SBSK*, 81–82.

69. Case 100, *SBSK*, 79–80.

70. Case 102, *SBSK*, 81–82. On fees paid to publicly hired caretakers in Niiya Village in Gunma prefecture in 1913, see "Seishinbyōsha toriatsukaihi kafu rinsei," in *Seishin shōgaisha mondai shiryō shūse*, ed. Okada Yasuo, Hashimoto Akira, and Komine Kazushige (Tokyo: Rikka shuppan, 2010–2011), 4:39–42.

71. Suzuki, "The State, Family, and the Insane in Japan," 202.

72. "Seishinbyōinhō seitei n ikan suru ken" (Naimu daijin, 1919), in *Seishin shōgaisha mondai shiryō shūse*, ed. Okada Yasuo, Hashimoto Akira, and Komine Kazushige (Tokyo: Rikka shuppan, 2010–2011), 4:184.

73. Akihito Suzuki, "Between Two Psychiatric Regimes: Migration and Psychiatry in Early Twentieth-Century Japan," in *Migration, Ethnicity, and Mental Health: International Perspectives, 1840–2010*, ed. Angela McCarthy and Catharine Coleborne (New York and London: Routledge, 2012), 147.

74. Suzuki, "Between Two Psychiatric Regimes," 149.

75. *SBSK*, 87–102.
76. Suzuki, "Between Two Psychiatric Regimes," 149.
77. Confinement in hospitals and homes shared architectural and spatial features, too, since national and prefectural ordinances and laws concerning home confinement drew from guidelines for building private confinement rooms within general and psychiatric hospitals. See Hashimoto, *Shitaku kanchi*, 34–39.
78. Both examples are from Ōji Brain Hospital case files from the late 1930s and early 1940s. Cited in Suzuki, "Between Two Psychiatric Regimes," 150–151.
79. Some psychiatrists criticized the Custody Law and other related prefectural ordinances for relying too heavily on the police for surveillance and data collection. Kure, for instance, argued that the police went as far as serving as substitutes for doctors in their interrogation of confined persons and their families about the nature and cause of the person's madness, as well as their individual and familial histories of illness. See *SBSK*, 126–127.

CHAPTER 3

1. The word 昆埪児 was used to refer to hypochondria, and 歇以私的里 was glossed in *furigana* as "heisuterii" (ヘイステリー). See Ogata Koan, *Fushi keiken ikun* vols. 1–25 (Osaka: Akitayataemon, 1857).
2. Like their counterparts elsewhere in the world, Japanese psychiatrists did not uniformly subscribe to a feminized understanding of hysteria. Psychiatrist Kure Shūzō's authoritative textbook of 1895, for instance, did not explain hysteria in gendered terms. Research on hysteria published in psychiatric and scientific journals in late nineteenth-century Japan, in fact, highlighted instances of male and child hysteria found in European clinical case studies. Japanese imperial army and navy health reports in the early twentieth century, too, documented diagnoses of hysteria among soldiers. See Sabine Frühstück, "Male Anxieities: Nerve Force, Nation, and the Power of Sexual Knowledge," *Journal of the Royal Asiatic Society* 15, no. 1 (April 2005): 77. On male hysteria in Europe and the United States, see Paul Lerner, *Hysterical Men: War, Psychiatry, and the Politics of Trauma in Germany, 1890–1930* (Ithaca, NY: Cornell University Press, 2003); Mark Micale, *Hysterical Men: The Hidden History of Male Nervous Illness* (Cambridge, MA: Harvard University Press, 2008).
3. Ishihara Chiaki, "Otoko wa shinkeisuijaku, onna wa hisuterii," *Hon* 31 (2006–2007): 34–41. For an overview of gendered notions of such neurological diseases as melancholy, hypochondria, and hysteria in European medical theories, see Elaine Showalter, "Hysteria, Feminism, and Gender," 286–344.
4. On neurasthenia, see, e.g., Junko Kitanaka, "Pathology of Overwork or Personality Weakness?: The Rise of Neurasthenia in Early-Twentieth-Century Japan," in *Depression in Japan: Psychiatric Cures for a Society in Distress* (Princeton, NJ: Princeton University Press, 2012), 54–66; Christopher Hill, "Exhausted by Their Battles with the World: Neurasthenia and Civilization Critique in Early-Twentieth-Century

Japan," in *Perversion and Modern Japan: Psychoanalysis, Literature, Culture*, ed. Nina Cornyetz and J. Keith Vincent (London and New York: Routledge, 2010), 242–258; Sabine Frühstück, "Male Anxieties: Nerve Force, Nation, and the Power of Sexual Knowledge," *Journal of the Royal Asiatic Society* 15, no. 1 (April 2005): 71–88; Watarai Yoshiichi, *Meiji no seishin isetsu: shinkeibyō shinkei suijaku kamigakari* (Tokyo: Iwanami shoten, 2003); Takahashi Masao, *Sōseki bungaku ga monogataru mono: shinkei suijakusha eno ikei to iyashi* (Tokyo: Misuzu shobō, 2009); Kawamura Kunimitsu, *Genshisuru kindai kūkan*. In contrast to neurasthenia, the topic of hysteria in early twentieth-century Japan has received relatively little sustained attention in Japanese or English. Two important exceptions include Satō Masahiro, *Seishin shikkan gensetsu no rekishi shakaigaku*; Mark Driscoll, "Empire in Hysterics," in *Absolute Erotic, Absolute Grotesque: The Living, Dead, and Undead in Japan's Imperialism, 1895–1945* (Durham: Duke University Press, 2010). The few studies on hysteria in Japanese are mostly about representations of hysteria in late-Meiji and Taisho novels, e.g., Izuhara Takatoshi, "Hisuterii—Mori Ōgai 'Hannichi,'" *Kokubungaku kaishaku to kyōzai no kenkyū* 46 (2001–2002): 185–187; Hibino Kei, "Hisuterii kanja to shite no Higuchi Ichiyō: Inoue Hisashi 'Zutsū katakori Higuchi Ichiyō' ron," *Kokubungaku kaishaku to kyōzai no kenkyū* 49 (2004–2008): 124–130; Egusa Mitsuko, "'Michikusa' no hisuterii," *Kokugo to kokubungaku* 851 (1994): 1–15.

5. Japanese male physicians and writers were not unique in using hysteria to create cultural narratives about the dangers of social change. Feminist histories of hysteria have shown how hysteria in nineteenth- and twentieth-century Western Europe and the United States marked off "realms of gendered cultural contestation" and was mobilized by physicians and others across time to denounce women's demands for expanded political and social roles. See Elaine Showalter, *Hystories: Hysterical Epidemics and Modern Culture* (New York: Columbia University Press, 1997). For first-generation feminist scholarship on hysteria in the 1970s, see Barbara Ehrenreich and Dierdre English, *Complaints and Disorders: The Sexual Politics of Sickness* (New York: The Feminist Press, 1973); Carroll Smith-Rosenberg, "The Hysterical Woman: Sex Roles and Role Conflict in Nineteenth Century America," *Social Research* 39 (Winter 1972): 652–678; Showalter, *The Female Malady*. For studies of hysteria informed by race theory and gender relations, see Briggs, "The Race of Hysteria"; Gail Bederman, *Manliness and Civilization: A Cultural History of Gender and Race in the United States, 1880–1917* (Chicago: University of Chicago Press, 1995); Gilman, "Black Bodies, White Bodies." For overviews of the historiography of hysteria, see Mark Micale, *Approaching Hysteria: Disease and Its Interpretations* (Princeton, NJ: Princeton University Press, 1995); Ilza Veith, *Hysteria: The History of a Disease* (Chicago: University of Chicago Press, 1965). Most studies of hysteria have focused on Europe and the United States, but important exceptions include Dikötter, *Sex, Culture, and Modernity in China*; Parle, *States of Mind*, 128–164.

6. On the purchase of daily newspapers and monthly magazines as the most rapidly expanding modern form of consumption, see Andrew Gordon, "Consumption,

Consumerism, and Japanese Modernity," in *The Oxford Handbook of the History of Consumption*, ed. Frank Trentmann (Oxford: Oxford University Press, 2012), 485–504. On women's magazines, see Sarah Frederick, *Turning Pages: Reading and Writing Women's Magazines in Interwar Japan* (Honolulu: University of Hawaii Press, 2006); Barbara Sato, *The New Japanese Woman: Modernity, Media, and Women in Interwar Japan* (Durham, NC: Duke University Press, 2003).

7. Das and Addlakha, "Disability and Domestic Citizenship."
8. Susan Burns, "Marketing Health and the Modern Body: Patent Medicine Advertisements in Meiji-Taishō Japan," in *East Asian Visual Culture from the Treaty Ports to World War II*, ed. Hans Thomsen and Jennifer Purtle (Chicago: Paragon Books, 2009), 176, 194. For patent medicine advertisements and pharmaceutical industries in the Japanese empire, see Hoi-eun Kim, "Cure for Empire: The 'Conquer-Russia-Pill,' Pharmaceutical Manufacturers, and the Making of Patriotic Japanese, 1904–45," *Medical History* 57, no. 2 (2013): 249–268; Hoi-eun Kim, "Adulterated Intermediaries: Peddlers, Pharmacists, and the Patent Medicine Industry in Colonial Korea (1910–1945)," *Enterprise & Society* 20, no. 4 (2019): 939–977; Timothy M. Yang, *A Medicated Empire*; Jin-kyung Park, "Managing 'Disease': Print Media, Medical Images, and Patent Medicine Advertisements in Colonial Korea," *International Journal of Cultural Studies* 21, no. 4 (2018): 420–439.
9. Burns, "Marketing Health," 177.
10. See Johnston, *The Modern Epidemic*; Susan Burns, *Kingdom of the Sick: A History of Leprosy and Japan* (Honolulu: University of Hawai'i Press, 2019).
11. Burns, "Marketing Health," 182.
12. Terazawa, *Knowledge, Power, and Women's Reproductive Health in Japan*; Aya Homei, "Birth Attendants in Meiji Japan."
13. Uno, "Womanhood, War, and Empire," 493; Jones, *Children as Treasures*, 121.
14. Sasaoka Shōzō, *Fujinbyōsha no kokoroe* (Tokyo: 1910), 1–2.
15. Margaret Lock, *Encounters with Aging: Mythologies of Menopause in Japan and North America* (Berkeley: University of California Press, 1993), 17. See also Satō Masahiro, *Seishin shikkan gensetsu no rekishi shakaigaku*, 190–199; Shirasugi Etsuo, "Hieshō no hakken," in *Kindai Nihon no shintai kankaku*, ed. Kuriyama Shigehisa and Kitazawa Kazutoshi (Tokyo: Seikyūsha, 2004), 65–68.
16. Matsumoto Ryōjun, *Minkan shobyō ryōchihō* (Tokyo: Shiseidō, 1880), 26–27.
17. Matsumoto Ryōjun, *Tsūzoku iryō benpō* (Kanagawa-ken: Chō Hideonori, 1892), 307–308.
18. The earliest references to hysteria after 1868 appeared in translations of American and European textbooks such as physician Kawada Kohei's (1836–1905) entry on hysteria in his translation of Henry Hartshorne's *Essentials of the Principles and Practice of Medicine* (1867 [translated 1872–1875]), Henry Hartshorne, *Naika tekiyō* (1872–1875), or *Essentials of the Principles and Practice of Medicine*, the first edition printed in Philadelphia in 1867. The entry on hysteria appears as one example of the larger category of "brain and nervous system disease." See Satō Masahiro, *Seishin shikkan gensetsu no rekishi shakaigaku*, 185.

19. Kure introduced the term "zōsōsho" (臓躁症) as the Japanese word for hysteria and refrained from including a *kana* gloss, which would indicate its pronunciation as *hisuterii*. Kure likely adapted the term "zōsō" from the Chinese medical classic *Essential Medical Treasures of the Golden Chamber* (*Kinki yōryaku hōron*), which featured an ailment called *fujin zōsō*, or "woman's mania" (婦人臓躁). According to the classic, women who suffered from *zōsō* were either flooded with a sadness that made them cry or were possessed by spirits. Yet Kure stripped the original Chinese term of the qualifier "fujin," or "women," briefly explaining at one point that both women and men could be afflicted by *zōsō*, though he admitted that young women between ages twenty and thirty, as well as children, both boys and girls around age ten, were disproportionally affected. See Kure Shūzō's *Seishinbyōgaku shūyō* (1895). On the origins of the term *zōsōsho*, see Ishii Atsushi, "Kamata Sekian *Fujin zōsōsetsu* kō," *Seishin igaku* 28, no. 5 (1986): 583–588.
20. *Yomiuri shinbun*, September 4, 1900, 6.
21. *Yomiuri shinbun*, January 12, 1900, 5.
22. *Yomiuri shinbun,* May 5, 1909, 4.
23. *Yomiuri shinbun*, August 29, 1910, 4.
24. *Yomiuri shinbun*, October 26, 1911, 4.
25. Harald Fuess, *Divorce in Japan: Family, Gender, and the State, 1600–2000* (Palo Alto, CA: Stanford University Press, 2004), 131; Isono Seichi and Isono Fujiko, *Kazoku seido* (Tokyo: Iwanami shinsho, 1958), 113; Yanagita Kunio, *Japanese Manners and Customs in the Meiji Era*, trans. Charles S. Terry (Tokyo: Ōbunsha, 1957), 169.
26. Tamura Kasaburō, *Shinkei no eisei* (Tokyo: Yomiuri shinbunsha, 1907), 110.
27. Tamura, *Shinkei*, 110.
28. Sugie Tadasu, *Hisuterii no kenkyū to sono ryōhō* (Tokyo: Shimada bunseikan, 1915), 1.
29. Many Japanese psychiatrists were influenced by neurologist Jean-Martin Charcot's work on hysteria at the Salpêtrière Hospital in Paris in the 1880s. Psychiatrist Miura Kinnosuke, for example, studied with Charcot for a few months in Paris and introduced the concept of "grande hystérie" (*dai hisuterii*) to Japan. See Motō Aki, "Sharukō no jidai to Miura Kinnosuke," *Rinshō shinkeigaku* 33 (1993): 1259–1264. Other psychiatrists, like Kure Shūzō, followed German-Austrian physician Richard von Krafft-Ebing's interpretations of hysteria more closely. See Kure, *Seishinbyōgaku shūyō* (Tokyo, 1895), 259–271.
30. Sugie, *Hisuterii no kenkyū*, 2.
31. Shimoda Mitsuzō and Sugita Naoki, *Saishin seishinbyōgaku* (Tokyo: Kokuseidō shoten, 1922), 412.
32. Credit is due to Suzuki Akihito for this formulation.
33. Cited in Donald Roden, "Taishō Culture and the Problem of Gender Ambivalence," in *Culture and Identity*, ed. Thomas Rimer (Princeton, NJ: Princeton University Press, 1990), 43.
34. Roden, "Taishō Culture," 44. See also Silverberg, *Erotic Grotesque Nonsense*.

35. Sugie, *Hisuterii no kenkyū*, 24.
36. Sugie and others were also reacting to new ideas about conjugal love circulating in the 1900s and 1910s. See Michiko Suzuki, *Becoming Modern Women: Love and Female Identity in Prewar Japanese Literature and Culture* (Stanford, CA: Stanford University Press, 2009).
37. Quoted in Jim Reichert, *In the Company of Men: Representations of Male-Male Sexuality in Meiji Literature* (Stanford, CA: Stanford University Press, 2006), 153.
38. Reichert, *In the Company of Men*, 173.
39. Sugie, *Hisuterii no kenkyū*, 25.
40. Sugie, *Hisuterii no kenkyū*, 33.
41. On police-sponsored personal consultation offices, see Margit Nagy, "'How Shall We Live?' Social Change, the Family Institution, and Feminism in Prewar Japan" (PhD diss., University of Washington, 1981), 175.
42. On the politics and science of male nervousness, see Frühstück, "Male Anxieties."
43. Women's involvement in the male-dominated world of mental healing was usually as subjects of hypnosis and other therapies that made male therapists famous. Kuwabara Toshirō, for instance, first experimented with hypnosis on a thirteen-year-old female servant in 1901, who showed signs of clairvoyance under hypnosis. The development of her extrasensory powers served as the basis upon which Kuwabara developed his then-famous theories of mind and religion. See Yoshinaga Shin'ichi, "The Birth of Japanese Mind Cure Methods," in *Religion and Psychotherapy in Modern Japan*, ed. Christopher Harding, Iwata Fumiaki, and Yoshinaga Shin'ichi (London: Routledge, 2015), 93.
44. Yu-chuan Wu, "A Disorder of Ki: Alternative Treatments for Neurasthenia in Japan, 1890–1945" (PhD diss., University College London, 2012), 172–175.
45. Yamano Haruo and Narita Ryūichi, "Minshū bunka to nashonarizumu," in *Kōza Nihonshi*, ed. Kenkyūkai Rekishigaku and Kenkyūkai Nihonshi (Tokyo: Tōkyō daigaku shuppankai, 1985): 9:253–292; Sheldon Garon, *Molding Japanese Minds: The State in Everyday Life* (Princeton, NJ: Princeton University Press, 1997), 82–83. On the appeal of New Religions among women and the relationship between such movements and gender, see Helen Hardacre, "Gender and the Millennium in Omotokyo, a Japanese New Religion," *Senri Ethnological Studies* 29 (January 1, 1990): 47–62; Helen Hardacre, *Kurozumikyō and the New Religions of Japan* (Princeton, NJ: Princeton University Press, 1986); Nancy K. Stalker, *Prophet Motive: Deguchi Onisaburō, Oomoto, and the Rise of New Religions in Imperial Japan* (Honolulu: University of Hawai'i Press, 2007).
46. See, e.g., Wu, "A Disorder of Ki"; Shimazono Susumu, *Iyasu chi no keifu: Kagaku to shūkyō no hasami* (Tokyo: Yoshikawa Kōbunkan, 2003).
47. The cost per day at Ōji Brain Hospital in Tokyo, for instance, was around 1.5 yen. A month-long stay would thus require a payment of 45 yen. In the 1920s, the typical starting monthly salaries for teachers was 40–45 yen, for bank clerks 50 yen, and

for civil servants 75 yen. Asashi Shinbunsha, ed., *Nedanshi nenpyo* (Tokyo: Asahi shinbunsha, 1988).

48. Burns, "Contemplating Places," 713–714.
49. Kawakami Takeshi, *Gendai nihon iryōshi* (Tokyo: Keisō Shobō, 1990), 67.
50. For evidence of the unevenness of the growth and distribution of doctors and hospitals, see Japan Statistical Association, ed., *Historical Statistics of Japan* (Tokyo: Statistics Bureau, Management and Coordination Agency, 1987–1988), 178–179 and 182–193.
51. For more on Iwakura, see Burns, "Reinvented Places."
52. Cited in Burns, "Contemplating Places," 708.
53. On the origins of such methods of observation and documentation in German academic psychiatry, see Akihito Suzuki, "Voices of Madness in Japan: Narrative Devices at the Psychiatric Bedside and in Modern Literature," in *The Routledge History of Madness and Mental Health*, ed. Greg Eghigian (London: Routledge, 2017), 245–260.
54. On historians' uses of psychiatric patient files, see Ana Antic, *Therapeutic Fascism: Experiencing the Violence of the Nazi New Order* (Oxford: Oxford University Press, 2016); Volker Hess and J. Andrew Mendelsohn, "Case and Series: Medical Knowledge and Paper Technology, 1600–1900," *History of Science* 48, no. 3–4 (2010): 287–314.
55. FO128 (1943/12/23 - 1944/4/11), Ōji Brain and Komine Hospital Archives, The Komine Institute, Tokyo, Japan.
56. For a set of drawings of monstrous spirits by a patient mostly likely admitted to Sugamo Hospital, see Kure Shūzō, *Seishin byōgaku shūyō* 1, ed. Haruo Akiyama (Tokyo: Sōzōshuppan, 2002 [1894]), insert between pages 26 and 27.
57. Suzuki, "Voices of Madness in Japan," 248–252.
58. Fukuda Mahito, ed., *Byōin to byōki* (Tokyo: Yumani Shobō, 2009).
59. Tomi Suzuki, *Narrating the Self: Fictions of Japanese Modernity* (Stanford, CA: Stanford University Press, 1996), 2.
60. Based on self-reported statistics in Nakamura Kokyō, *Seishineisei kōwa*, 3 vols. (Shufu no tomo sha, 1933).
61. Morita and Nakamura belonged to a circle of doctors, writers, literary critics, legal scholars, criminologists, and others who collaborated across disciplinary boundaries to investigate the workings of the human psyche from the 1910s to 1930s. Many contributed to the journal founded by Nakamura in 1915, *Hentai shinri*, which published articles on psychopathology, criminal psychology, forensic medicine, and sex education not only by doctors, but also by influential critics and political theorists, including Abe Isoo, Yoshino Sakuzō, Hasegawa Nyozekan, and Ikuta Chōkō. Nakamura also founded the Society for Japanese Psychiatry in 1916, to which Morita and others belonged. Members of the society traveled together to conduct experiments on *nensha*, or thoughtography, and

attended lectures on the practice of Tairedo. See Oda Susumu, *"Hentai shinri" to Nakamura Kokyō.*

62. Nakamura Kokyō, "Shinkeisuijaku ya hisuterii wa dō sureba zenchi suru ka," *Shufu no tomo* 12, no. 10 (1928): 240–244; 12, no. 11 (1928): 188–192; 12, no. 12 (1928): 228–232; 13, no. 1 (1929): 272–277; Nakamura Kokyō, *Hisuterii no ryōhō* (Tokyo: Shufu no tomo sha, 1932).

63. Nakamura, "Ryōyōhō no jyunjo," *Hisuterii no ryōhō.*

64. On Buddhist influences on Japanese psychotherapy in the early twentieth century, especially Morita Masatake's therapy, see, e.g., Kondo Kyoichi and Kitanishi Kenji, "The Mind and Healing in Morita Therapy," in *Religion and Psychotherapy in Modern Japan*, 103–119.

65. Example 2 in Nakamura, *Hisuterii no ryōhō*, 195–198.

66. Nakamura, *Hisuterii no ryōhō*, 199.

67. Nakamura, *Hisuterii no ryōhō*, 206.

68. Nakamura, *Hisuterii no ryōhō*, 205.

69. Akihito Suzuki, "Disorderly Women in the Family: Analysis of Female Patients at a Psychiatric Hospital in Tokyo c. 1920–1945," paper presentation, Johns Hopkins University, November 1, 2016.

70. Nakamura, *Hisuterii no ryōhō*, 116.

71. Nakamura, *Hisuterii no ryōhō*, 217.

72. On the early modern origins of the idea that personal cultivation leads to social, physical, and material well-being, see, e.g., Janine Sawada, *Practical Pursuits: Religion, Politics, and Personal Cultivation in Nineteenth-Century Japan* (Honolulu: University of Hawai'i Press, 2004).

CHAPTER 4

1. Case 3, "Hysterical Personality—Menstrual Psychosis—Murder," in Kominami Mataichirō, *Hōigaku tanpenshū*, Kindai Hanzai Kagaku Zenshū 8 (Tokyo: Bukyōsha, 1930), 465–487.

2. Ornella Moscucci, *The Science of Woman: Gynaecology and Gender in England, 1800–1929* (Cambridge: Cambridge University Press, 1990); Roth, *A Miscarriage of Justice*; Constance Backhouse, "Desperate Women and Compassionate Courts: Infanticide in Nineteenth-Century Canada," *University of Toronto Law Journal* 34 (1984): 447–478; Marland, *Dangerous Motherhood.*

3. For instance, Cassia Roth shows how judicial leniency in cases of "reproductive crimes" such as abortion and infanticide in turn-of-the-twentieth-century Rio de Janeiro resulted from the judicial system's infantilization of women, as seen in its refusals to prosecute women for having committed such crimes. Other historians of Latin America have argued that nineteenth-century legal systems incorporated "honor clauses" that allowed women to invoke honor as the motive for a crime and therefore receive a reduced sentence. See Roth, *A Miscarriage of Justice,*

181–207; Nora E. Jaffary, "Reconceiving Motherhood: Infanticide and Abortion in Colonial Mexico," *Journal of Family History* 37, no. 1 (2012): 3–22; Kristin Ruggiero, "Honor, Maternity, and the Disciplining of Women: Infanticide in Late Nineteenth-Century Buenos Aires," *Hispanic American Historical Review* 72, no. 3 (1992): 353–373; Laura Shelton, "Bodies of Evidence: Honor, *Prueba Plena*, and Emerging Medical Discourses in Northern Mexico's Infanticide Trials in the Late Nineteenth and Early Twentieth Centuries," *Americas* 74, no. 4 (2017): 457–480. On British and related contexts, see Arlie Loughnan, *Manifest Madness: Mental Incapacity in the Criminal Law* (Oxford: Oxford University Press, 2012); Wendy Chan, Dorothy E. Chunn, and Robert Menzies, eds., *Women, Madness, and the Law: A Feminist Reader* (London: Glass House, 2005).

4. On judicial leniency for those considered mad in the Edo period, see Hiruta Genshirō, "Nihon ni okeru seishin shōgaisha no sekinin nōryoku to kango ni kansuru hōseido," *Seishin shinkei gaku zasshi* 105, no. 2 (2003): 187–193.

5. The diagnosis known as "menstrual psychosis" (*gekkei seishinbyō*) was made famous by Austrian–German psychiatrist Richard von Krafft-Ebing in 1902 when he published an article and a monograph on the subject with forty-seven observations of women who were hospitalized or who had committed crimes under the influence of the disorder. The diagnosis was not universally accepted, since many of his contemporaries believed the symptoms had less to do with menstruation and more with hereditary factors. In Japan, menstrual psychosis was not a standardized term. Many Japanese psychiatrists and criminologists referred to the condition as menstruation-induced "mental abnormality" (*seishin ijō*). See Richard von Krafft-Ebing, "Psychosis Menstrualis: eine klinisch-forensische Studie" (Stuttgart: Enke, 1902); Ian Brockington, "Menstrual Psychosis," *World Psychiatry* 4, no. 1 (2005): 1–9; Tanaka Hikaru, *Gekkei to hanzai: josei hanzairon no shingi wo tou* (Tokyo: Hihyōsha, 2006), 14–17.

6. Veronika Fuechtner, Douglas E. Haynes, and Ryan M. Jones, eds., *A Global History of Sexual Science, 1880–1960* (Berkeley: University of California Press, 2017); Durba Mitra, *Indian Sex Life: Sexuality and the Colonial Origins of Modern Social Thought* (Princeton, NJ: Princeton University Press, 2020); and Frühstück, *Colonizing Sex*.

7. Such moments evoke the ways in which psychiatry and family often "leaned" on one another. See Michel Foucault, *Psychiatric Power* (New York: Picador, 2008), 94.

8. Similar tensions and collusions arose between law and psychiatry in societies across the world, especially in cases involving the criminalization of certain forms and acts of sexuality ("sexual psychopathy"). See Susan R. Schmeiser, "The Ungovernable Citizen: Psychopathy, Sexuality, and the Rise of Medico-Legal Reasoning," *Yale Journal of Legal History* 20, no. 2 (2008): 163–240,. See also Philomena Mariani, "Law-and-Order Science," in *Constructing Masculinity*, eds Maurice Berger, Brian Wallis, and Simon Watson (New York: Routledge, 1995), 135–156.

9. Röhl, ed., *History of Law in Japan since 1868*, 611.

10. Article 64 in French Penal Code of 1810: "Il n'y a ni crime ni délit, lorsque le prévenu était en état de démence au temps de l'action, ou lorsqu'il a été contraint par une force à laquelle il n'a pu resister." See *Kyū keihō: Meiji 13-nen*, ed. Nishihara Haruo et al. (Tokyo: Shinzansha, 1994–1997).

11. *Hōrei zensho* (Tokyo: Naikaku kanpōkyō, 1880), 101.

12. The following remarks by Katayama are cited in Nagai Junko, "'Seishinbyōsha' to keihō dai sanjūkyūjyō no seiritsu," *Soshio saiensu* 11 (2005), 230–233.

13. The fourth kind of person was referred to as a "borderline person" (*chūkansha*), or someone who was neither completely healthy nor sick, but fell somewhere in the middle. See Hyōdō, *Seishinbyō no nihon kindai*, 203–207.

14. Nagai, "'Seishinbyōsha' to keihō," 233.

15. Nagai, "'Seishinbyōsha' to keihō," 235.

16. Law no. 45 in *Hōrei zensho* 2 (1907), 67; "*Keihō*" in Japanese Ministry of Justice's Japanese Law Translation Database System, http://www.japaneselawtranslation. go.jp.

17. Kure Shūzō, "Seishinbyōsha to shinkeihō," *Keijihō hyōrin* (October 1909), 13. Also cited in Serizawa, *"Hō" kara kaihōsareru kenryoku*, 110.

18. Yamane Masatsugu, "Seishinbyō gakka setchi ni kan suru kengian," *Shinkeigaku zasshi* (April 1906): 53.

19. Jennifer Robertson, "Shingaku Woman: Straight from the Heart," in *Recreating Japanese Women, 1600–1945*, ed. Gail Lee Bernstein (Berkeley: University of California Press, 1991), 91.

20. Diana E. Wright, "Female Crime and State Punishment in Early Modern Japan," *Journal of Women's History* 16, no. 3 (2004): 17.

21. Christine L. Marran, *Poison Woman: Figuring Female Transgression in Modern Japanese Culture* (Minneapolis: University of Minnesota Press, 2007), 22. See also Shimizu Shōjirō, *Meiji, Taishō, Shōwa norowareta josei hanzai* (Tokyo: Yoshie Shobō, 1965).

22. Frühstück, *Colonizing Sex*; Oda Makoto, *Sei* (Tokyo: Sanseidō, 1996); Nina Cornyetz and J. Keith Vincent, eds., *Perversion and Modern Japan: Psychoanalysis, Literature, Culture* (New York: Routledge, 2010); Gregory Pflugfelder, *Cartographies of Desire: Male-Male Sexuality in Japanese Discourse, 1600–1950* (Berkeley: University of California Press, 1999); Oosterhuis, *Stepchildren of Nature*.

23. Cited in Marran, *Poison Woman*, 115. The textual crime wave consisted of the publication of journals such as *Criminology* (Hanzai Kagaku), *Criminal Journal* (Hanzai Kōron), *True Stories of Crime* (Hanzai Jitsuwa), *The True Story Times* (Jitsuwa Jidai), and *Criminology Research* (Hanzai Kagaku Kenkyū), as well as the sixteen-volume *Collected Works of Modern Criminology* (Kinda Kagaku Zenshū) (Tokyo: Bukyōsha, 1929–1930).

24. The notion first appeared in Cesare Lombroso, *Uomo delinquente* (1876). For an English translation, see Cesare Lombroso, *Criminal Man*, trans. Mary Gibson and Nicole Hahn Rafter (Durham, NC: Duke University Press, 2006).

25. In later editions of his work, Lombroso modified his teaching by allowing that born criminals accounted for only about a third of all criminals and by explaining the born criminal in terms of mental illness rather than as an atavistic throwback to primitive man, but his conviction that the born criminal was an anthropological type with distinct physical characteristic remained unchanged. See Richard Wetzell, "Criminology in Weimar and Nazi Germany," in *Criminals and Their Scientists: The History of Criminology in International Perspective*, ed. Peter Becker and Richard F. Wetzell (Cambridge: Cambridge University Press, 2009), 402.

26. See Richard Wetzell, *Inventing the Criminal: A History of German Criminology, 1880–1945* (Chapel Hill: University of North Carolina Press, 2000). On the creation across Europe of a penal regime emphasizing the criminal rather than the criminal offense, potential dangerousness rather than actual harm, see Michel Foucault, "Truth and Juridical Forms," in *Power*, ed. James D. Faubion; trans. Robert Hurley et al. (New York: New Press, 2000), 56–57, and "About the Concept of the 'Dangerous Individual' in Nineteenth-Century Legal Psychiatry," trans. Alain Baudot and Jane Couchman, *International Journal of Law and Psychiatry* 1 (1978): 1–18.

27. Cited in Hyōdō, *Seishinbyō no nihon kindai*, 200. See also Serizawa, *"Hō" kara kaihōsareru kenryoku*, 23–84.

28. Yoji Nakatani, "The Birth of Criminology in Modern Japan," in *Criminals and Their Scientists: The History of Criminology in International Perspective*, ed. Peter Becker and Richard F. Wetzell (Cambridge: Cambridge University Press, 2009), 287. See also Minoru Shikita and Shinichi Tsuchiya, *Crime and Criminal Policy in Japan: Analysis and Evaluation of the Showa Era, 1926–1988* (New York: Springer-Verlag, 1992).

29. On "erotic grotesque nonsense" culture, see, e.g., Silverberg, *Erotic Grotesque Nonsense*; Mark Driscoll, *Absolute Erotic, Absolute Grotesque: The Living, Dead, and Undead in Japan's Imperialism, 1895–1945* (Durham, NC: Duke University Press, 2010).

30. Of course, female criminality and transgression was a source of anxiety in places other than Japan as well at the turn of the twentieth century. See, e.g., Ann-Louise Shapiro, *Breaking the Code: Female Criminality in Fin-de-Siècle Paris* (Stanford, CA: Stanford University Press, 1996); Lisa Duggan, *Sapphic Slashers: Sex, Violence, and American Modernity* (Durham, NC: Duke University Press, 2001). On the construction of sexuality as a dangerous drive that formed the core of new such identities as "the menstruating girl" and "the hysterical housewife," see Dikötter, *Sex, Culture, and Modernity in China*.

31. Habuto Eiji and Sawada Junjirō, *Hanzai no kenkyū* (Tokyo: Hōbundō Shoten, 1916), 356.

32. Izumi Nakayama, "Periodic Struggles: Menstruation Leave in Japan" (PhD diss., Harvard University, 2007).

33. Kaneko Junji, *Hanzaisha no shinri*, Kindai hanzai kagaku zenshū (Tokyo: Bukyōsha, 1930), 100–101.

34. Nozoe Atsuyoshi, *Josei to hanzai*, Kindai hanzai kagaku zenshū (Tokyo: Bukyōsha, 1930), 1.

35. Contemporaries in Germany were making similar arguments in the 1920s. Medical doctor Erich Wulffen wrote in his *Woman as Sexual Criminal* that "woman is a born sexual criminal" and that "most of woman's criminal tendencies, on account of close lying psycho-physiological causes, stand in some fixed relation to her sex life. In this sense then, the female thief, swindler, extortionist, incendiary, robber, murderer, may be regarded as a sexual criminal." Cited in Marran, *Poison Woman*, 118 and 120.

36. Cited in Tanaka, *Gekkei to hanzai*, 87.

37. Kure Shūzō and Katayama Kunika, *Hōigaku taisei* (Tokyo: Shūnan shoin, 1895). See Yamagami Akira, "Seishin kantei—sono rekishiteki hensen to shomondai," *Seishin igaku* 41, no. 10 (1999): 1032–1042.

38. Kure Shūzō and Sakaki Hajime, *Hōigaku teikō* (Tokyo: Kure Shūzō, 1897).

39. See Yamagami, "Seishin kantei," 1032.

40. Kure Shūzō, *Seishinbyō kanteirei*, vols. 1–4 (Tokyo: Tohōdō, 1903–1909).

41. Kure Shūzō and Sakaki Hajime, *Hōigaku teikō*, 3:5. Forensic medicine and medical jurisprudence developed on a global scale in the late nineteenth and early twentieth centuries. See, e.g., Daniel Asen, *Death in Beijing: Murder and Forensic Science in Republican China* (Cambridge: Cambridge University Press, 2016); Michael Clark and Catherine Crawford, *Legal Medicine in History* (Cambridge: Cambridge University Press, 1994); Joel Peter Eigen, *Unconscious Crime: Mental Absence and Criminal Responsibility in Victorian London* (Baltimore: Johns Hopkins University Press, 2004).

42. On the rise of detective fiction in Japan, see, e.g., Yoshida Morio, *Tantei shōsetsu to nihon kindai* (Tokyo: Seikyūsha, 2004); Uchida Ryūzō, *Tantei shōsetsu no shakaigaku* (Tokyo: Iwanami shoten, 2001); Satoru Saito, *Detective Fiction and the Rise of the Japanese Novel, 1880–1930* (Cambridge, MA: Harvard University Asia Center, 2012); Sari Kawana, *Murder Most Modern: Detective Fiction and Japanese Culture* (Minneapolis: University of Minnesota Press, 2008); Mark Silver, *Purloined Letters: Cultural Borrowing and Japanese Crime Literature, 1868–1937* (Honolulu: University of Hawai'i Press, 2008).

43. See Kathryn Montgomery Hunter, *Doctors' Stories: The Narrative Structure of Medical Knowledge* (Princeton, NJ: Princeton University Press, 1991), 52.

44. Kominami Mataichirō, *Hōigaku tanpenshū*. Forensic psychiatric reports submitted to district-level courts can be found in a range of sources. Many reports were published by individual psychiatrists in academic medical journals, official collections of mental evaluations (*kanteisho shū*), and popular journals. Some appeared in abridged form in publications on women and crime, including the aforementioned *Modern Criminology* series of 1929–1930.

45. Jordan Sand and Steven Wills, "Governance, Arson, and Firefighting in Edo, 1600–1868," in *Flammable Cities: Urban Conflagration and the Making of the Modern World*, ed. Greg Bankoff, Uwe Luebken, and Jordan Sand (Madison: University of Wisconsin Press, 2012), 47.

46. Case 4, "Hysterical Idiocy—Menstrual Psychosis—Arson," in *Hōigaku tanpenshū*, 495.

47. Satō, *Seishin shikkan gensetsu no rekishi shakaigaku*, 82–84.

48. Keiko Daidoji, "What a Household with Sick Persons Should Know," 184–185.

49. Case 4, "Hysterical Idiocy—Menstrual Psychosis—Arson," in *Hōigaku tanpenshū*, 503.

50. Case 4, "Hysterical Idiocy," 497.

51. Case 6, "Manic-depressive Disorder (*sōutsukyō*)—Person with Excitable Temperament—Responsible Agent," 523–228.

52. Case 5, "A Person of Diminished Competence—Menstrual Psychosis—Arson," 509.

53. Case 6, "Manic–depressive Disorder," 539.

54. Case 6, "Manic–depressive Disorder," 547.

55. Case 6, "Manic–depressive Disorder," 546.

56. Case 6, "Manic–depressive Disorder," 530.

57. Case 6, "Manic–depressive Disorder," 533.

58. *Jiji shinpō,* December 27, 1916. See Tanaka, *Gekkei to hanzai*, 16.

59. Tanaka, *Gekkei to hanzai*, 14.

60. Kamichika's imprisonment and crime became a public scandal and was widely reported in newspapers. Her story was also the inspiration for the postwar film *Eros Plus Massacre* (1969).

61. Case 1, "Temporary Mental Abnormality during Menstruation—Attempted Murder," *Hōigaku tanpenshū*, 423–447.

62. Case 1, "Temporary Mental Abnormality," 441.

63. Case 1, "Temporary Mental Abnormality," 440.

64. Most studies of working-class women of the early twentieth century focus on factory workers in the textile industry, white collar female workers in cities, and employees of service-based urban jobs. Far less attention has been paid to women without permanent work who might be called itinerants. See Janet Hunter, ed., *Japanese Women Working* (London: Routledge, 1993). One exception is writer and poet Hayashi Fumiko's self-portrayal as an itinerant woman in her novel *Diary of a Vagabond* (1930). See Joan Ericson, *Be a Woman: Hayashi Fumiko and Modern Japanese Women's Literature* (Honolulu: University of Hawai'i Press, 1997).

65. Scholarship on Abe Sada is extensive. See, e.g., William Johnston, *Geisha, Harlot, Strangler, Star: A Woman, Sex, and Morality in Modern Japan* (New York: Columbia University Press, 2005); Marran, *Poison Woman*, 103–135.

66. Marran, *Poison Woman*, 111.

EPILOGUE: POSTWAR CULTURES OF GENDERED CARE
AND KINSHIP

1. See, e.g., Eguchi Shigeyuki, "Between Folk Concepts of Illness and Psychiatric Diagnosis: *Kitsune-tsuki* (Fox Possession) in a Mountain Village of Western Japan," *Culture, Medicine, and Psychiatry* 15 (1991): 421–451; Matsuoka Etsuko, "The Interpretations of Fox Possession: Illness as Metaphor," *Culture, Medicine,*

and Psychiatry 15 (1991): 453–477; Teigo Yoshida, "Mystical Retribution, Spirit Possession, and Social Structure in a Japanese Village," *Ethnology* 6 (July 1967): 237–262; Teigo Yoshida, "Spirit Possession and Village Conflict," in *Conflict in Japan,* ed. Ellis S Krauss, Thomas Rohlen, and Patricia Steinhoff (Honolulu: University of Hawai'i Press, 1984), 85–104.

2. The Mental Hygiene Law (Seishin Eisei Hō) of 1950 banned home confinement, but the practice did not disappear. Home confinement in postwar Okinawa, for instance, has recently captured much public attention. See Hashimoto Akira, "Seishinbyōsha kangōhō ka no Okinawa (1900–1960 nen) to shitake kanchi," *Shakai fukushi kenkyū* 22 (2020): 21–38; Kyosuki Yamamoto, "Woman's Search for Grandfather Reveals 'Home Custody' System," *The Asahi Shimbun*, March 13, 2021, https://www.asahi.com/ajw/articles/14172616; *Yoake mae no uta: kesareta Okinawa no shōgaisha*, directed by Hara Yoshikazu (Shōgaisha eizō bunka kenkyūjo Image Satellite, 2020), 97 mins.

3. On the history of eugenics in Japan, see, e.g., Yōko Matsubara, "The Enactment of Japan's Sterilization Laws in the 1940s: A Prelude to Postwar Eugenic Policy," *Historia Scientiarum* 8, no. 2 (December 1998): 187–201; Fujime Yuki, *Sei no rekishigaku* (Tokyo: Fuji Shuppan, 1997); Suzuki Zenji, *Nihon no yūseigaku* (Tokyo: Sankyō Shuppan, 1983); Sumiko Otsubo, "Engendering Eugenics: Feminists and Marriage Restriction Legislation in the 1920s," in *Gendering Modern Japanese History*, ed. Barbara Molony and Kathleen S. Uno (Cambridge, MA: Harvard University Asia Center, 2005): 225–256; Suzuki Zenji, Matsubara Yōko, and Sakano Tōru, "Yūseigaku-shi kenkyū no dōkō III: Amerika oyobi Nihon no yūseigaku ni kansuru rekishi kenkyū," *Kagakushi kenkyū* 34 (1995): 101–106.

4. Matsubara, "The Enactment of Japan's Sterilization Laws."

5. Janice Matsumura, "Eugenics, Environment, and Acclimatizing to Manchukuo: Psychiatric Studies of Japanese Colonists," *Nihon ishigaku zasshi* 56, no. 3 (2010): 329–350.

6. Matsubara, "The Enactment of Japan's Sterilization Laws."

7. On the passage of the Mental Hygiene Law (Seishin Eisei Hō) of 1950, see Janice Matsumura, "Mental Health as Public Peace: Kaneko Junji and the Promotion of Psychiatry in Modern Japan," *Modern Asian Studies* 38, no. 4 (2004): 899–930.

8. Matsumura, "Mental Health as Public Peace," 922. Psychiatric hospitals were overcrowded, with occupancy at 112 percent (36,969 patients for 32,834 beds) in 1954, according to a 1960 Ministry of Health and Welfare report. Cited in Karen Nakamura, *A Disability of the Soul: An Ethnography of Schizophrenia and Mental Illness in Contemporary Japan* (Ithaca, NY: Cornell University Press, 2013), 48.

9. Nakamura, *Disability of the Soul*, 47–48.

10. Despo Kritsotaki, Vicky Long, and Matthew Smith, eds., *Deinstitutionalisation and After* (Cham: Palgrave Macmillan: 2016).

11. Matsumura, "Mental Health as Public Peace," 922.

12. Nakamura, *Disability of the Soul*, 53–69.

13. A 2003 government survey of people with registered psychiatric disabilities living outside of hospitals showed that 76.8 percent lived with family. Others lived alone (17.9 percent), in welfare homes (1.3 percent), in group homes (1.7 percent), and in elderly nursing homes (0.5 percent). The remaining patients (1.8%) were not residing in any of the above places. Cited in Nakamura, *Disability of the Soul*, 69.

14. Patients, families, and activists have long advocated for alternatives to hospital-based care such as independent living and small group home facilities. Yet in Japan and elsewhere, the shift from hospital-based care to so-called community care has relocated patients simply to settings other than the hospital, including the streets, transportation depots, prisons, and hostile neighborhoods. See Anne M. Lovell and Nancy Scheper-Hughes, "Deinstitutionalization and Psychiatric Expertise: Reflections on Dangerousness, Deviancy, and Madness," *International Journal of Law and Psychiatry* 9 (1986): 361–381.

15. See, e.g., Tsunetsugu Munakata, "Japanese Attitudes toward Mental Illness and Mental Health Care," in *Japanese Culture and Behavior*, ed. Takie Sugiyama Lebra and William P. Libra (Honolulu: University of Hawai'i Press, 1986), 369–378. Some scholars have argued that auxiliary help from families has enabled Japanese psychiatric hospitals to maintain a lower ratio of professionals to patients, thereby reducing costs. See Kiyoka Koizumi and Paul Harris, "Mental Health Care in Japan," *Hospital and Community Psychiatry* 43, no. 11 (November 1992): 1102.

16. On family-provided care within hospitals, see Graham Mooney and Jonathan Reinarz, eds., *Permeable Walls: Historical Perspectives on Hospital and Asylum Visiting* (Amsterdam: Rodopi, 2009).

17. Garon, "State and Family in Modern Japan," 323.

18. See, e.g., Andrew Gordon, "Managing the Japanese Household: The New Life Movement in Postwar Japan," *Social Politics* 4, no. 2 (1997): 245–283.

19. Garon, "State and Family in Modern Japan," 330.

20. Amy Borovoy, *The Too-Good Wife: Alcohol, Codependency, and the Politics of Nurturance in Postwar Japan* (Berkeley: University of California Press, 2005), 20; Andrew Gordon, "Managing the Japanese Household"; Suzanne Vogel, *Professional Housewife: The Career of Urban Middle Class Japanese Women* (Cambridge, MA: Institute for Independent Study, Radcliffe College, 1988).

21. Sheldon Garon, "State and Family in Modern Japan."

22. Borovoy, *The Too-Good Wife*, 20. On the "around the body care" performed by women, see Takie Lebra, *Japanese Women: Constraint and Fulfillment* (Honolulu: University of Hawaii Press, 1984).

23. Borovoy, *The Too-Good Wife*, 21.

24. Eiko Shinotsuka, "Japanese Care Assistants in Hospitals, 1918–1988," in *Japanese Women Working*, ed. Janet Hunter (London: Routledge, 1993), 149–180.

25. William Caudill, "Around the Clock Patient Care in Japanese Psychiatric Hospitals: The Role of the Tsukisoi," *American Sociological Review* 26, no. 2 (1961): 204–214.

26. Caudill, "Around the Clock Patient Care in Japanese Psychiatric Hospitals," 205. There is a rich anthropological literature on "motherly" roles and cultures of dependency that helped create essentialist notions of "Japanese-ness" in the postwar period. See, e.g., Amy Borovoy, "Doi Takeo and the Rehabilitation of Particularism in Postwar Japan," *Journal of Japanese Studies* 38, no. 2 (2012): 263–295.

27. Goldfarb, " 'Coming to Look Alike' "; Goldfarb, "Beyond Blood Ties."

28. Amy Borovoy, "Japan's Hidden Youths: Mainstreaming the Emotionally Distressed in Japan," *Culture, Medicine, and Psychiatry* 32, no. 4 (2008): 566.

29. Borovoy, "Japan's Hidden Youths," 554.

30. Satō, *Seishin shikkan gensetsu no rekishi shakaigaku*, 319–412.

31. John Dower, "Peace and Democracy in Two Systems," in *Postwar Japan as History*, ed. Andrew Gordon (Berkeley: University of California Press, 1993), 17.

32. Nancy Rosenberger, "Middle-aged Japanese Women and the Meanings of the Menopausal Transition" (PhD diss., University of Michigan, 1984); Nancy Rosenberger, "Productivity, Sexuality, and Ideologies of Menopausal Problems in Japan," in *Health, Illness, and Medical Care in Japan: Cultural and Social Dimensions*, ed. Edward Norbeck and Margaret Lock (Honolulu: University of Hawai'i Press, 1987), 158–188.

33. Margaret M. Lock, *Encounters with Aging: Mythologies of Menopause in Japan and North America* (Berkeley: University of California Press, 1993), 19.

34. See, e.g., Christopher Burton, ed., *ABC of Medically Unexplained Symptoms* (New York: John Wiley & Sons, 2012).

35. Akaeda Hideo, Akaeda Yuichi, and Akaeda Tsuneo, *Shirarezaru fujinbyō futei shūso* (Tokyo: Fujin seikatsusha, 1980). Cited in Margaret Lock, "Protests of a Good Wife and Wise Mother: The Medicalization of Distress in Japan," in *Health, Illness, and Medical Care in Japan: Cultural and Social Dimensions*, ed. Edward Norbeck and Margaret Lock (Honolulu: University of Hawai'i Press, 1987), 126.

36. Nancy R. Rosenberger, "The Process of Discourse: Usages of a Japanese Medical Term," *Social Science and Medicine* 34 (1992): 237–247.

37. Lock, "Protests of a Good Wife and Wise Mother," 244.

38. Kitanaka, *Depression in Japan*, 142.

39. Kitanaka, *Depression in Japan*, 142.

40. Kitanaka, *Depression in Japan*, 142.

41. Lock, "Protests of a Good Wife and Wise Mother," 138.

42. Ito Peng, "Social Care in Crisis: Gender, Demography, and Welfare State Restructuring in Japan," *Social Politics* 9, no. 3 (2002): 411–443.

43. Patricia Boling, "State Feminism in Japan?" *U.S.-Japan Women's Journal* 34 (2008): 68–89. On the backlash against gender equity policies in the 2000s, see Tomomi Yamaguchi, "The Mainstreaming of Feminism and the Politics of Backlash in Twenty-First-Century Japan," in *Rethinking Japanese Feminisms*, ed. Julia C. Bullock, Ayako Kano, and James Walker (Honolulu: University of Hawai'i Press, 2017), 68–85.

Bibliography

Akaeda, Hideo, Akaeda Yuichi, and Akaeda Tsuneo. *Shirarezaru fujinbyō futei shūso*. Tokyo: Fujin Seikatsusha, 1980.

Akakura, Takako. "Meiji 33 nen 'Seishinbyōsha kangohō' no mondaiten to shinhō seiritsu ni mukete no katsudō: Taishō 8 nen 'Seishinbyōinhō' seiritsu no haikei." *Rokkōdai ronshū* 47, no. 3 (2001): 1–69.

Akimasa, Miyake. "Female Workers of the Urban Lower Class." In *Technology Change and Female Labour in Japan*, edited by Masanori Nakamura, 97–131. Tokyo: United Nations Press, 1994.

Ambros, Barbara. "Clerical Demographics in the Edo-Meiji Transition: Shingon and Tōzanha Shugendō in Western Sagami." *Monumenta Nipponica* 64 (2009): 83–125.

Antic, Ana. *Therapeutic Fascism: Experiencing the Violence of the Nazi New Order*. Oxford: Oxford University Press, 2016.

Aoyama, Yōji. "Seishinbyōsha no kazoku no yakuwari: seishinbyōsha kangōhō ni yoru kanri shisutemuu." *Kaihō shakaigaku kenkyū* 14 (2000): 116–133.

Araki, Sōtarō. "Tokushimakenka no inugamitsuki oyobi tanukitsuki ni tsuite." *Chūgai iji shinpō* 485 (June 5, 1900): 5–12.

Asahi, Shinbunshi, ed. *Nedanshi nenpyō*. Tokyo: Asahi Shinbunsha, 1988.

Asen, Daniel. *Death in Beijing: Murder and Forensic Science in Republican China*. Cambridge: Cambridge University Press, 2016.

Aulino, Felicity. *Rituals of Care: Karmic Politics in an Aging Thailand*. Ithaca, NY: Cornell University Press, 2019.

Austin, Michael R. *Negotiating with Imperialism: The Unequal Treaties and the Culture of Japanese Diplomacy*. Cambridge, MA: Harvard University Press, 2006.

Backhouse, Constance. "Desperate Women and Compassionate Courts: Infanticide in Nineteenth-Century Canada." *University of Toronto Law Journal* 34 (1984): 447–478.

Baelz, Erwin. *Awakening Japan: The Diary of a German Doctor*. Translated by Eden Paul and Cedar Paul. New York: Viking Press, 1932.

Baelz, Erwin. "Kohyō byōsetsu." *Iji shinbun*, no. 148 (1885).

Bartlett, Peter, and David Wright, eds. *Outside the Walls of the Asylum: The History of Care in the Community, 1750–2000*. New Brunswick, NJ: The Athlone Press, 1999.

Bathgate, Michael. *The Fox's Craft in Japanese Religion and Folklore: Shapeshifters, Transformations, and Duplicities*. New York and London: Routledge, 2004.

Baum, Emily. *The Invention of Madness: State, Society, and the Beijing Insane, 1900–1937*. Chicago: University of Chicago Press, 2018.

Baum, Emily, and Howard Chiang, eds. "Histories and Cultures of Mental Health in Modern East Asia: New Directions." *History of the Behavioral Sciences* 57, no. 3 (Summer 2021): 239–242.

Bederman, Gail. *Manliness and Civilization: A Cultural History of Gender and Race in the United States, 1880–1917*. Chicago: University of Chicago Press, 1995.

Behringer, Wolfgang. *Shaman of Oberstdorf: Chonrad Stoeckhlin and the Phantoms of the Night*. Charlottesville: University Press of Virginia, 1998.

Bernstein, Gail. "Women in the Silk-Reeling Industry in Nineteenth Century Japan." In *Japan and the World: Essays on Japanese History and Politics in Honour of Ishida Takeshi*, edited by Gail Lee Bernstein and Haruhiro Fukui, 54–77. London: Palgrave Macmillan, 1988.

Berry, Mary Elizabeth, and Marcia Yonemoto, eds. *What Is a Family?: Answers from Early Modern Japan*. Berkeley: University of California Press, 2019.

Blacker, Carmen. *The Catalpa Bow: A Study of Shamanistic Practices in Japan*. London: Allen & Unwin, 1975.

Bledsoe, Caroline. *Contingent Lives: Fertility, Time, and Aging in West Africa*. Chicago: University of Chicago Press, 2002.

Boling, Patricia. "State Feminism in Japan?" *U.S.-Japan Women's Journal* 34 (2008): 68–89.

Borovoy, Amy. "Doi Takeo and the Rehabilitation of Particularism in Postwar Japan." *Journal of Japanese Studies* 38, no. 2 (2012): 263–295.

Borovoy, Amy. "Japan's Hidden Youths: Mainstreaming the Emotionally Distressed in Japan." *Culture, Medicine, and Psychiatry* 32, no. 4 (2008): 552–576.

Borovoy, Amy. *The Too-Good Wife: Alcohol, Codependency, and the Politics of Nurturance in Postwar Japan*. Berkeley: University of California Press, 2005.

Botsman, Daniel. *Punishment and Power in the Making of Modern Japan*. Princeton, NJ: Princeton University Press, 2007.

Brecher, W. Puck. *The Aesthetics of Strangeness: Eccentricity and Madness in Early Modern Japan*. Honolulu: University of Hawai'i Press, 2013.

Briggs, Laura. "The Race of Hysteria: 'Overcivilization' and the 'Savage' Woman in Late Nineteenth-Century Obstetrics and Gynecology." *American Quarterly* 52, no. 2 (2000): 246–273.

Briggs, Robin. *Witches and Neighbors: The Social and Cultural Context of European Witchcraft*. New York: Penguin Books, 1998.

Brockington, Ian. "Menstrual Psychosis." *World Psychiatry* 4, no. 1 (2005): 1–9.

Brooks, Barbara J. "Japanese Colonialism, Gender, and Household Registration: Legal Reconstruction of Boundaries." In *Gender and Law in the Japanese Imperium*, edited by Susan L. Burns and Barbara J. Brooks, 219–239. Honolulu: University of Hawai'i Press, 2013.

Brown, Kathleen. *Foul Bodies: Cleanliness in Early America*. New Haven, CT: Yale University Press, 2011.

Burns, Susan. "Bodies and Borders: Syphilis, Prostitution, and the Nation in Japan, 1860–1890." *U.S.-Japan Women's Journal*. English Supplement 15 (1998): 3–30.

Burns, Susan. "Constructing the National Body: Public Health and the Nation in Nineteenth-Century Japan." In *Nation Work: Asian Elites and National Identities*, edited by Timothy Brook and Andre Schmid, 17–28. Ann Arbor: University of Michigan Press, 2000.

Burns, Susan. "Contemplating Places: The Hospital as Modern Experience in Meiji Japan." In *New Directions in the Study of Meiji Japan*, edited by Helen Hardacre and Adam L. Kern, 702–718. Leiden: Brill, 1997.

Burns, Susan. *Kingdom of the Sick: A History of Leprosy and Japan*. Honolulu: University of Hawai'i Press, 2019.

Burns, Susan. "Marketing Health and the Modern Body: Patent Medicine Advertisements in Meiji-Taishō Japan." In *East Asian Visual Culture from the Treaty Ports to World War II*, edited by Hans Thomsen and Jennifer Purtle, 173–196. Chicago: Paragon Books, 2009.

Burns, Susan. "Nanayama Jundō at Work: A Village Doctor and Medical Knowledge in Nineteenth Century Japan." *East Asian Science, Technology, and Medicine* 29 (2008): 62–83.

Burns, Susan. "Reinvented Places: 'Tradition,' 'Family Care' and Psychiatric Institutions in Japan." *Social History of Medicine* 32 (February 2019): 99–120.

Burns, Susan. "Relocating Psychiatric Knowledge: Meiji Psychiatrists, Local Culture(s), and the Problem of Fox Possession." *Historia Scientiarum* 22, no. 2 (December 2012): 88–109.

Butler, Judith. *Antigone's Claims: Kinship between Life and Death*. New York: Columbia University Press, 2000.

Caudill, William. "Around the Clock Patient Care in Japanese Psychiatric Hospitals: The Role of the Tsukisoi." *American Sociological Review* 26, no. 2 (1961): 204–214.

Chakrabarty, Dipesh. *Provincializing Europe: Postcolonial Thought and Historical Difference*. Princeton, NJ: Princeton University Press, 2000.

Chamberlain, Basil Hall. *Things Japanese: Being Notes on Various Subjects Connected with Japan for the Use of Travellers and Others*. London; Yokohama; Shanghai: John Murray; Kelly & Walsh, 1905.

Chan, Wendy, Dorothy E. Chunn, and Robert Menzies, eds. *Women, Madness, and the Law: A Feminist Reader*. London: Glass House, 2005.

Chen Chao-ju, "*Sim-pua* under the Colonial Gaze: Gender, 'Old Customs,' and the Law in Taiwan under Japanese Imperialism." In *Gender and Law in the*

Japanese Imperium, edited by Susan L. Burns and Barbara J. Brooks, 189–218. Honolulu: University of Hawai'i Press, 2013.

Chen, Hsiu-fen. "Between Passion and Repression: Medical Views of Demon Dreams, Demonic Fetuses, and Female Sexual Madness in Late Imperial China." *Late Imperial China* 32, no. 1 (June 2011): 51–82.

Chua, Jocelyn Lim. *In Pursuit of the Good Life: Aspiration and Suicide in Globalizing South India*. Berkeley: University of California Press, 2014.

Clark, Michael, and Catherine Crawford. *Legal Medicine in History*,. Cambridge: Cambridge University Press, 1994.

Clark, Stuart. *Thinking with Demons: The Idea of Witchcraft in Early Modern Europe*. Oxford: Clarendon Press, 1997.

Clark, Stuart, ed. *Languages of Witchcraft: Narrative, Ideology and Meaning in Early Modern Culture*. New York: St. Martin's Press, 2001.

Cornyetz, Nina, and J. Keith Vincent, eds. *Perversion and Modern Japan: Psychoanalysis, Literature, Culture*. New York: Routledge, 2010.

Daidoji, Keiko. "Treating Emotion-Related Disorders in Japanese Traditional Medicine: Language, Patients and Doctors." *Culture, Medicine, and Psychiatry* 37 (March 2013): 59–80.

Daidoji, Keiko. *What a Household with Sick Persons Should Know: Expressions of Body and Illness in a Medical Text of Early Nineteenth-Century Japan*. PhD diss., University of London, 2009.

Das, Debjani. *House of Madness: Insanity and Asylums of Bengal in Nineteenth-Century India*. New Delhi: Oxford University Press, 2015.

Das, Veena. *Affliction: Health, Disease, Poverty*. New York: Fordham University Press, 2015.

Das, Veena, and Renu Addlakha. "Disability and Domestic Citizenship: Voice, Gender, and the Making of the Subject." *Public Culture* 13, no. 3 (2001): 511–531.

Dikötter, Frank. *Sex, Culture, and Modernity in China: Medical Science and the Construction of Sexual Identities in the Early Republican Period*. Hong Kong: Hong Kong University Press, 1995.

Dower, John. "Peace and Democracy in Two Systems." In *Postwar Japan as History*, edited by Andrew Gordon, 305–492. Berkeley: University of California Press, 1993.

Driscoll, Mark. *Absolute Erotic, Absolute Grotesque: The Living, Dead, and Undead in Japan's Imperialism, 1895–1945*. Durham, NC: Duke University Press, 2010.

Duggan, Lisa. *Sapphic Slashers: Sex, Violence, and American Modernity*. Durham, NC: Duke University Press, 2001.

Edington, Claire. *Beyond the Asylum: Mental Illness in French Colonial Vietnam*. Ithaca, NY: Cornell University Press, 2019.

Eguchi, Shigeyuki. "Between Folk Concepts of Illness and Psychiatric Diagnosis: *Kitsune-Tsuki* (Fox Possession) in a Mountain Village of Western Japan." *Culture, Medicine, and Psychiatry* 15 (1991): 421–451.

Egusa, Mitsuko. " 'Michikusa' no hisuterii." *Kokugo to kokubungaku* 851 (1994): 1–15.

Ehlers, Maren. *Give and Take: Poverty and the Status Order in Early Modern Japan.* Cambridge, MA: Harvard University Asia Center, 2018.

Ehrenreich, Barbara, and Dierdre English. *Complaints and Disorders: The Sexual Politics of Sickness.* New York: The Feminist Press, 1973.

Eigen, Joel Peter. *Unconscious Crime: Mental Absence and Criminal Responsibility in Victorian London.* Baltimore: Johns Hopkins University Press, 2004.

El Shakry, Omnia. *The Arabic Freud: Psychoanalysis and Islam in Modern Egypt.* Princeton, NJ: Princeton University Press, 2017.

Elman, Benjamin. "Sinophiles and Sinophobes in Tokugawa Japan: Politics, Classicism, and Medicine during the Eighteenth Century." *East Asian Science, Technology and Society* 2, no. 1 (2008): 93–121.

Ericson, Joan. *Be a Woman: Hayashi Fumiko and Modern Japanese Women's Literature.* Honolulu: University of Hawai'i Press, 1997.

Faison, Elyssa. *Managing Women: Disciplining Labor in Modern Japan.* Berkeley: University of California Press, 2007.

Fielder, Brigitte. *Relative Races: Genealogies of Interracial Kinship in Nineteenth-Century America.* Durham, NC: Duke University Press, 2020.

Figal, Gerald. *Civilization and Monsters: Spirits of Modernity in Meiji Japan.* Durham, NC: Duke University Press, 1999.

Fissell, Mary. "Women, Health, and Healing in Early Modern Europe." *Bulletin of the History of Medicine* 82, no. 1 (2008): 1–17.

Foster, Michael Dylan. "Haunting Modernity: Tanuki, Trains, and Transformation in Japan." *Asian Ethnology* 71, no. 1 (2012): 3–29.

Foster, Michael Dylan. *Pandemonium and Parade: Japanese Monsters and the Culture of Yōkai.* Berkeley: University of California Press, 2009.

Foucault, Michel. "About the Concept of the 'Dangerous Individual' in Nineteenth-Century Legal Psychiatry." Translated by Alain Baudot and Jane Couchman. *International Journal of Law and Psychiatry* 1 (1978): 1–18.

Foucault, Michel. *Psychiatric Power.* New York: Picador, 2008.

Foucault, Michel. "Truth and Juridical Forms." In *Power,* edited by James D. Faubion, translated by Robert Hurley, 1–89. New York: New Press, 2000.

Frederick, Sarah. *Turning Pages: Reading and Writing Women's Magazines in Interwar Japan.* Honolulu: University of Hawai'i Press, 2006.

Freedman, Alisa, Laura Miller, and Christine R. Yano, eds. *Modern Girls on the Go: Gender, Mobility, and Labor in Japan.* Palo Alto, CA: Stanford University Press, 2013.

Frühstück, Sabine. *Colonizing Sex: Sexology and Social Control in Modern Japan.* Berkeley: University of California Press, 2003.

Frühstück, Sabine. "Male Anxieties: Nerve Force, Nation, and the Power of Sexual Knowledge." *Journal of the Royal Asiatic Society* 15, no. 1 (April 2005): 71–89.

Fuechtner, Veronika, and Douglas E. Haynes, eds. *A Global History of Sexual Science, 1880–1960.* Berkeley: University of California Press, 2017.

Fuess, Harald. *Divorce in Japan: Family, Gender, and the State, 1600–2000*. Palo Alto, CA: Stanford University Press, 2004.

Fujime, Yuki. *Sei no rekishigaku*. Tokyo: Fuji Shuppan, 1997.

Fujitani, James. "The Jesuit Hospital in the Religious Context of Sixteenth-Century Japan." *Japanese Journal of Religious Studies* 46, no. 1 (2019): 79–101.

Fukuda, Mahito, ed. *Byōin to byōki*. Tokyo: Yumani Shobō, 2009.

Fukushima, Masao. "Meiji yonen kosei hō no shiteki zentei to sono kōzō." In *Kosei seido to "ie" seido*, edited by Masao Fukushima, 94–169. Tokyo: Tokyo Daigaku Shuppankai, 1959.

Furth, Charlotte. *A Flourishing Yin: Gender in China's Medical History, 960–1665*. Berkeley: University of California Press, 1999.

Garcia, Angela. *The Pastoral Clinic: Addiction and Dispossession along the Rio Grande*. Berkeley: University of California Press, 2010.

Garon, Sheldon. *Molding Japanese Minds: The State in Everyday Life*. Princeton, NJ: Princeton University Press, 1997.

Garon, Sheldon. "State and Family in Modern Japan: A Historical Perspective." *Economy and Society* 39, no. 3 (2010): 317–336.

Gaskill, Malcolm. "The Pursuit of Reality: Recent Research into the History of Witchcraft." *Historical Journal* 51, no. 4 (2008): 1069–1088.

Gilman, Sander. "Black Bodies, White Bodies: Toward an Iconography of Female Sexuality in Late Nineteenth-Century Art, Medicine, and Literature." *Critical Inquiry* 12, no. 1 (1985): 204–242.

Gluck, Carol. *Japan's Modern Myths: Ideology in the Late Meiji Period*. Princeton, NJ: Princeton University Press, 1985.

Goble, Andrew Edmund. "Women and Medicine in Late 16th Century Japan: The Example of the Honganji Religious Community in Osaka and Kyoto as Recorded in the Diary of Physician Yamashina Tokitsune." *Asia Pacific Perspectives* 14, no. 1 (2016): 51–52.

Goldfarb, Kathryn E. "Beyond Blood Ties: Intimate Kinships in Japanese Foster and Adoptive Care." In *Intimate Japan: Ethnographies of Closeness and Conflict*, edited by Alison Alexy and Emma E. Cook, 181–198. Honolulu: University of Hawai'i Press, 2018.

Goldfarb, Kathryn E. "'Coming to Look Alike': Materializing Affinity in Japanese Foster and Adoptive Care." *Social Analysis* 60, no. 2 (Summer 2016): 47–64.

Gordon, Andrew. "Consumption, Consumerism, and Japanese Modernity." In *The Oxford Handbook of the History of Consumption*, edited by Frank Trentmann, 485–504. Oxford: Oxford University Press, 2012.

Gordon, Andrew. "Managing the Japanese Household: The New Life Movement in Postwar Japan." *Social Politics* 4, no. 2 (1997): 245–283.

Grapard, Allan G. "Japan's Ignored Cultural Revolution: The Separation of Shinto and Buddhist Divinities in Meiji ("Shimbutsu Bunri") and a Case Study: Tōnomine." *History of Religions* 23, no. 3 (1984): 240–265.

Habuto, Eiji, and Sawada Junjirō. *Hanzai no kenkyū.* Tokyo: Hōbundō Shoten, 1916.

Han, Clara. *Seeing Like a Child: Inheriting the Korean War.* New York: Fordham University Press, 2021.

Hanson, Marta. "Depleted Men, Emotional Women: Gender and Medicine in the Ming Dynasty." *NAN NÜ* 7, no. 2 (January 1, 2005): 287–304. https://doi.org/10.1163/156852605775248694.

Hardacre, Helen. "Conflict between Shugendō and the New Religions of Bakumatsu Japan." *Japanese Journal of Religious Studies* 21, no. 2/3 (September 1994): 137–166.

Hardacre, Helen. "Gender and the Millennium in Ōmotokyō, a Japanese New Religion." *Senri Ethnological Studies* 29 (1990): 47–62.

Hardacre, Helen. *Kurozumikyō and the New Religions of Japan.* Princeton, NJ: Princeton University Press, 1986.

Harding, Christopher, Fumiaki Iwata, and Shin'ichi Yoshinaga, eds. *Religion and Psychotherapy in Modern Japan.* Abingdon: Routledge, 2015.

Hashimoto, Akira. *Chiryō no basho to seishin iryōshi.* Tokyo: Nihon Hyōronsha, 2010.

Hashimoto, Akira. "Seishinbyōsha kangohōka no Okinawa (1900–1960) to shitakukanchi: Okinawaken kōbunshokan shozō shiryō no bunseki." *Shakai fukushi kenkyū* 22 (2020): 21–38.

Hashimoto, Akira. *Seishinbyōsha to shitaku kanchi.* Tokyo: Rikka Shuppan, 2011.

Hayami, Akira. "The Myth of Primogeniture and Impartible Inheritance in Tokugawa Japan." *Journal of Family History* 8 (1983): 3–28.

Hayami, Yasutaka. *Tsukimono-mochi meishin: sono rekishiteki kōsatsu.* Tokyo: Akashi Shoten, 1999.

Hess, Volker, and J. Andrew Mendelsohn. "Case and Series: Medical Knowledge and Paper Technology, 1600–1900." *History of Science* 48, no. 3–4 (2010): 287–314.

Hibino, Kei. "Hisuterii kanja to shite no Higuchi Ichiyō: Inoue Hisashi 'Zutsū katakori Higuchi Ichiyō' ron." *Kokubungaku kaishaku to kyōzai no kenkyū* 49 (2004–2008): 124–130.

Hill, Christopher. "Exhausted by Their Battles with the World: Neurasthenia and Civilization Critique in Early-Twentieth-Century Japan." In *Perversion and Modern Japan: Psychoanalysis, Literature, Culture,* edited by Nina Cornyetz and J. Keith Vincent, 242–258. London and New York: Routledge, 2010.

Hiroshi, Yasui. *Berutsu no shōgai: kindai igaku dōnyū no chichi.* Kyoto: Shinbunkaku, 1995.

Hirota, Masaki. *Sabetsu no shosō. Nihon kindai shisō taikei.* Edited by Shūichi Katō. Vol. 22. Tokyo: Iwanami Shoten, 1990.

Hiruta, Genshirō. *Hayariyamai to kitsunetsuki: kinsei shomin no iryō jijō.* Tokyo: Misuzi Shobō, 1985.

Hiruta, Genshirō. "Japanese Psychiatry in the Edo Period (1600–1868)." *History of Psychiatry* 13 (2002): 131–151.

Hiruta, Genshirō. "Nihon ni okeru seishin shōgaisha no sekinin nōryoku to kango ni kansuru hōseido." *Seishin shinkei gaku zasshi* 105, no. 2 (2003): 187–193.

Hofmann-Kuroda, Lisa. *The Tree of Life: The Politics of Kinship in Meiji Japan (1870–1915)*. PhD diss., University of California Berkeley, 2018.

Hōgetsu, Rie. *Kindai nihon ni okeru eisei no tenkai to juyō*. Tokyo: Tōshindō, 2010.

Homei, Aya. "'Seijō san' to 'Kindai eisei': Kindai sanba no senmon bunya wo meguru poritikkusu." *Seibutsugaku shi kenkyū* 70 (December 2002): 1–16.

Honda, Yoshiharu, Suzuki, Hideo, Honda, Hideharu, and Irisawa, Satoshi. "Chihō toshi seishinbyōin ni okeru sagyōryōhō no kusawake." *Seishin shinkeigaku zasshi* 111, no. 9 (2009): 1047–1054.

Hōrei Zensho. Tokyo: Naikaku Kanpōkyō, 1887–1912.

Hozumi, Yatsuka. "Minpō idete, chūkō horobu." In *Meiji shisō shū 2*, Vol. 31. Kindai Nihon shisō taikei. Tokyo: Chikuma Shobō, 1977: 391–394.

Hunter, Janet. *Women and the Labour Market in Japan's Industrialising Economy: The Textile Industry before the Pacific War*. London: Routledge Curzon, 2003.

Hunter, Janet, ed. *Japanese Women Working*. London: Routledge, 1993.

Hunter, Kathryn Montgomery. *Doctors' Stories: The Narrative Structure of Medical Knowledge*. Princeton, NJ: Princeton University Press, 1991.

Hyōdō, Akiko. *Seishinbyō no nihon kindai: tsuku shinshin kara yamu shinshin e*. Tokyo: Seikyūsha, 2008.

Ikegami, Yoshimasa. "Local Newspaper Coverage of Folk Shamans in Aomori Prefecture." In *Folk Beliefs in Modern Japan*, edited by Nobutaka Inoue, 9–91. Tokyo: Kokugakuin University, 1994.

Illouz, Eva. *Saving the Modern Soul: Therapy, Emotions, and the Culture of Self-Help*. Berkeley: University of California Press, 2008.

Ishihara, Chiaki. "Otoko wa shinkeisuijaku, onna wa hisuterii." *Hon* 31 (2006–2007): 34–41.

Ishii, Atsushi. "Kamata Sekian Fujin zōsōsetsu kō." *Seishin igaku* 28, no. 5 (1986): 583–588.

Ishii, Ryōsuke. *Nihon sōzokuhō shi*. Tokyo: Sōbunsha, 1980.

Ishikawa, Tadashi. "Human Trafficking and Intra-Imperial Knowledge: Adopted Daughters, Households, and Law in Imperial Japan and Colonial Taiwan." *Journal of Women's History* 29, no. 3 (2017): 37–60.

Ishizuka, Takatoshi. *Nihon no tsukimono: zokushin wa ima mo ikite iru*. Tokyo: Miraisha, 1972.

Isono, Seichi, and Isono, Fujiko. *Kazoku seidō*. Tokyo: Iwanami Shinsho, 1958.

Itahara, Kazuko, and Kuwabara, Haruo. "Edo jidai koki ni okeru seishin shōgai no shogu III." *Shakai mondai kenkyū* 49, no. 2 (2000): 183–200.

Itahara, Kazuko, and Kuwabara, Haruo. "Edo jidai koki ni okeru seishin shōgai no shogu IV." *Shakai mondai kenkyū* 50 (2000): 80.

Ito, Ken. *An Age of Melodrama: Family, Gender, and Social Hierarchy in the Turn-of-the-Century Japanese Novel*. Stanford, CA: Stanford University Press, 2008.

Itō, Mikiharu. *Kazoku kokkakan no jinruigaku*. Kyoto: Mineruva Shobō, 1982.

Izuhara, Takatoshi. "Hisuterii—Mori Ōgai 'Hannichi.'" *Kokubungaku kaishaku to kyōzai no kenkyū* 46 (February 2001): 185–187.

Jaffary, Nora E. "Reconceiving Motherhood: Infanticide and Abortion in Colonial Mexico." *Journal of Family History* 37, no. 1 (2012): 3–22.

Jannetta, Ann Bowman. *The Vaccinators: Smallpox, Medical Knowledge, and the 'Opening' of Japan*. Stanford, CA: Stanford University Press, 2007.

Japan Statistical Association, ed. *Historical Statistics of Japan*. Tokyo: Japan Statistical Association, 1987.

Jiji Shinpō, 1912–1916.

Johnson, Jessica Marie. *Wicked Flesh: Black Women, Intimacy, and Freedom in the Atlantic World*. Philadelphia: University of Pennsylvania Press, 2020.

Johnston, William. "Buddhism contra Cholera: How the Meiji State Recruited Religion against Epidemic Disease." In *Science, Technology, and Medicine in the Modern Japanese Empire*, edited by David G. Wittner and Philip C. Brown, 62–78. London: Routledge, 2016.

Johnston, William. *Geisha, Harlot, Strangler, Star: A Woman, Sex, and Morality in Modern Japan*. New York: Columbia University Press, 2005.

Johnston, William. *The Modern Epidemic: A History of Tuberculosis in Japan*. Cambridge, MA: Council on East Asian Studies, Harvard University, 1995.

Jones, Mark. *Children as Treasures: Childhood and the Middle Class in Early Twentieth Century Japan*. Cambridge, MA: Harvard University Asia Center, 2010.

Josephson, Jason Ananda. *The Invention of Religion in Japan*. Chicago: University of Chicago Press, 2012.

Kadowaki, Sakae. *Kōhyōbyō shinron*. Tokyo: Sōzō Shuppan, 2001 [1902].

Kanekawa, Hideo. *Seishinbyōin no shakaishi*. Tokyo: Seikyūsha, 2009.

Kaneko, Junji. *Hanzaisha No Shinri, Kindai Hanzai Kagaku Zenshū*. Tokyo: Bukyōsha, 1930.

Kasahara, Hidehiko, and Kojima, Kazutaka. *Meiji-ki iryō eisei gyōsei no kenkyū*. Kyoto: Mineruva Shobō, 2011.

Katakura, Hisako, Nagahara, Kazuo, and Yoshie, Akiko. "Edo machikata ni okeru sōzoku." In *Sōzoku to kasan*, 89–112. Tokyo: Yoshikawa Kōbunkan, 2003.

Katsu, Kokichi. *Musui dokugen: hoka*. Tokyo: Heibonsha, 1969 [1843].

Kawahara, Yukiko. *Local Development in Japan: The Case of Shimane Prefecture from 1800–1930*. PhD diss., University of Arizona, 1990.

Kawakami, Takeshi. *Gendai nihon iryōshi*. Tokyo: Keisō Shobō, 1990.

Kawamura, Kunimitsu. *Genshi suru kindai kūkan: meishin, byōki, zashikirō, aruiwa rekishi no kioku*. Tokyo: Seikyūsha, 1990.

Kawamura, Kunimitsu. *Hyōi no kindai to poritikusu*. Tokyo: Seikyūsha, 2007.

Kawana, Sari. *Murder Most Modern: Detective Fiction and Japanese Culture*. Minneapolis: University of Minnesota Press, 2008.

Kawashima, Takeyoshi. *Ideorogii to shite no kazoku seido*. Tokyo: Iwanami Shoten, 1957.

Kayaoğlu, Turan. *Legal Imperialism: Sovereignty and Extraterritoriality in Japan, the Ottoman Empire and China*. Cambridge: Cambridge University Press, 2010.

Ketelaar, James. *Of Heretics and Martyrs in Meiji Japan: Buddhism and Its Persecution.* Princeton, NJ: Princeton University Press, 1993.

Kim, Hoi-eun. "Adulterated Intermediaries: Peddlers, Pharmacists, and the Patent Medicine Industry in Colonial Korea (1910–1945)." *Enterprise & Society* 20, no. 4 (2019): 939–977.

Kim, Hoi-eun. "Cure for Empire: The 'Conquer-Russia-Pill,' Pharmaceutical Manufacturers, and the Making of Patriotic Japanese, 1904–45." *Medical History* 57, no. 2 (2013): 249–268.

Kim, Hoi-eun. *Doctors of Empire: Medical and Cultural Encounters between Imperial Germany and Meiji Japan.* Toronto: University of Toronto Press, 2014.

Kim, Sonja M. *Imperatives of Care: Women and Medicine in Colonial Korea.* Honolulu: University of Hawai'i Press, 2019.

Kim, Yumi. "Seeing Cages: Home Confinement in Early Twentieth-Century Japan." *Journal of Asian Studies* 77, no. 3 (2018): 635–658.

Kitamura, Harumatsu. *Seishinbyōsha kangohōrei jimon jitō roku.* Osaka: Keisatsubu, 1904.

Kitamura, Ryōtaku. "Tohō ron (1817)." In *Iseidō sōsho,* edited by Shūzō Kure. Kyoto: Shinbunkaku, 1970 [1923]: 39–53.

Kitanaka, Junko. *Depression in Japan: Psychiatric Cures for a Society in Distress.* Princeton, NJ: Princeton University Press, 2012.

Kitanaka, Junko. "The Rebirth of Secrets and the New Care of the Self in Depressed Japan." *Current Anthropology* 56, supp. 12 (December 2015): 251–262.

Kleinman, Arthur. "Caregiving: The Divided Meaning of Being Human and the Divided Self of the Caregiver." In *Rethinking the Human,* edited by J. Michelle Molina, Donald K Swearer, and Susan Lloyd McGarry, 17–31. Cambridge, MA: Center for the Study of World Religions, Harvard Divinity School, 2010.

Kleinman, Arthur. *The Illness Narratives: Suffering, Healing, and the Human Condition.* New York: Basic Books, 1988.

Kleinman, Arthur. *The Soul of Care: The Moral Education of a Husband and Doctor.* New York: Viking, 2019.

Kobayashi, Takehiro. *Kindai nihon to koshū eisei.* Tokyo: Yūzankaku, 2001.

Koizumi, Kiyoka, and Paul Harris. "Mental Health Care in Japan." *Hospital and Community Psychiatry* 43, no. 11 (November 1992): 1100–1103.

Komatsu, Kazuhiko. *Hyōrei shinkōro.* Tokyo: Hatsubaisho Gendai Jānarizumu Shuppankai, 1982.

Kominami, Mataichirō. *Hōigaku tanpenshū.* Kindai Hanzai Kagaku Zenshū 8. Tokyo: Bukyōsha, 1930.

Kōnusuke, Odaka. "Redundancy Utilized: The Economics of Female Domestic Servants in Pre-War Japan." In *Japanese Women Working,* edited by Janet Hunter, 16–36. London: Routledge, 1993.

Koyama, Shizuko. *Ryōsai kenbo to iu kihan.* Tokyo: Keisō Shobō, 1991.

Krafft-Ebing, Richard von. *Lehrbuch der Psychiatrie auf klinischer Grundlage für praktische Ärzte und Studierende.* 3rd ed. Stuttgart: Verlag von Ferdinand Enke, 1888.

Krafft-Ebing, Richard von. *Psychosis menstrualis: Eine klinisch-forensische Studie.* Stuttgart: Enke, 1902.

Krafft-Ebing, Richard von. *Textbook of Insanity Based on Clinical Observations for Practitioners and Students of Medicine.* Translated by Charles Gilbert Chaddock. London: F. A. Davis Company, 1904.

Kritsotaki, Despo, Vicky Long, and Matthew Smith, eds. *Deinstitutionalisation and After.* Cham: Palgrave Macmillan, 2016.

Kure, Shūzō. "Kōhyōbyō to 'hisuterii' to no kankei." *Katei eisei sōsho* 4 (1905): 63–79.

Kure, Shūzō. *Seishin byōsha shitaku kanchi no jikkyō.* Tokyo: Naimushō Eiseikyoku, 1918.

Kure, Shūzō. *Seishinbyō kanteirei.* 4 vols. Tokyo: Tohōdō, 1903.

Kure, Shūzō. *Seishinbyōgaku shūyō.* Tokyo, 1895.

Kure, Shūzō, and Kashida, Gorō. *Seishin byōsha shitaku kanchi no jitsujyō oyobi sono tōkeiteki kansatsu.* Tokyo: Sōzō Shuppan, 2000 [1918].

Kure, Shūzō, and Kashida, Gorō. "Seishinbyōsha shitaku kanchi no jikkyō oyobi sono tōkeiteki kansatsu." *Tōkyō igakukai zasshi* 32, no. 10–13 (1918): 521–715.

Kure, Shūzō, and Katayama, Kunika. *Hōigaku taisei.* Tokyo: Shūnan shoin, 1895.

Kure, Shūzō, and Katayama, Kunika. *Hōigaku teikō.* Tokyo: Kure Shūzō, 1897.

Lambe, Jennifer. *Madhouse: Psychiatry and Politics in Cuban History.* Chapel Hill: University of North Carolina Press, 2017.

Laugier, Sandra. "The Ethics of Care as a Politics of the Ordinary." *New Literary History* 46, no. 2 (2015): 217–240.

Lebra, Takie. *Japanese Women: Constraint and Fulfillment.* Honolulu: University of Hawai'i Press, 1984.

Lerner, Paul. *Hysterical Men: War, Psychiatry, and the Politics of Trauma in Germany, 1890–1930.* Ithaca, NY: Cornell University Press, 2003.

Libbrecht, Katrien. *Hysterical Psychosis: A Historical Survey.* New Brunswick, NJ: Transaction Publishers, 1995.

Lim, Sungyun. *Rules of the House: Family Law and Domestic Disputes in Colonial Korea.* Berkeley: University of Calfironia Press, 2019.

Lock, Margaret. *Encounters with Aging: Mythologies of Menopause in Japan and North America.* Berkeley: University of California Press, 1993.

Lock, Margaret. "Protests of a Good Wife and Wise Mother: The Medicalization of Distress in Japan." In *Health, Illness, and Medical Care in Japan: Cultural and Social Dimensions,* edited by Edward Norbeck and Margaret Lock, 115–144. Honolulu: University of Hawai'i Press, 1987.

Loh, Kah Seng. "Mental Illness in Singapore: A History of a Colony, Port City, and Coolie Town." *East Asian Science, Technology, and Society* 10, no. 2 (2016): 121–140.

Lombroso, Cesare. *Criminal Man.* Translated by Mary Gibson and Nicole Hahn Rafter. Durham, NC: Duke University Press, 2006.

Lönholm, Ludwig. *The Civil Code of Japan.* Tokyo: Kokubunsha, 1898.

Loughnan, Arlie. *Manifest Madness: Mental Incapacity in the Criminal Law.* Oxford: Oxford University Press, 2012.

Lovell, Anne M., and Nancy Scheper-Hughes. "Deinstitutionalization and Psychiatric Expertise: Reflections on Dangerousness, Deviancy, and Madness." *International Journal of Law and Psychiatry* 9 (1986): 361–381.

Lunbeck, Elizabeth. *The Psychiatric Persuasion: Knowledge, Gender, and Power in Modern America*. Princeton, NJ: Princeton University Press, 1994.

Ma, Zhiying. "Madness, Architecture, and the Built Environment: Psychiatric Spaces in Historical Context." In *Psychiatry and Chinese History*, edited by Howard Chiang, 91–110. London: Routledge, 2015.

Mariani, Philomena. "Law-and-Order Science." In *Constructing Masculinity*, edited by Maurice Berger, Brian Wallis, and Simon Watson, 135–156. New York: Routledge, 1995.

Marland, Hilary. *Dangerous Motherhood: Insanity and Childbirth in Victorian Britain*. New York: Palgrave Macmillan, 2004.

Marran, Christine L. *Poison Woman: Figuring Female Transgression in Modern Japanese Culture*. Minneapolis: University of Minnesota Press, 2007.

Martin, Emily. *The Woman in the Body: A Cultural Analysis of Reproduction*. Boston: Beacon Press, 1987.

Matsubara, Yōko. "The Enactment of Japan's Sterilization Laws in the 1940s: A Prelude to Postwar Eugenic Policy." *Historia Scientiarum* 8, no. 2 (December 1998): 187–201.

Matsumoto, Ryōjun. *Minkan shobyō ryōchihō*. Tokyo: Shiseidō, 1880.

Matsumoto, Ryōjun. *Tsūzoku iryō benpō*. Kanagawa: Chō Hideonori, 1892.

Matsumura, Janice. "Eugenics, Environment, and Acclimatizing to Manchukuo: Psychiatric Studies of Japanese Colonies." *Nihon Ishigaku Zasshi* 56, no. 3 (2010): 329–350.

Matsumura, Janice. "State Propaganda and Mental Disorders: The Issue of Psychiatric Casualties among Japanese Soldiers during the Asia-Pacific War." *Bulletin of the History of Medicine* 78, no. 4 (Winter 2004): 804–835.

Matsuoka, Etsuko. "The Interpretations of Fox Possession: Illness as Metaphor." *Culture, Medicine, and Psychiatry* 15 (1991): 453–477.

Maxey, Trent E. *The "Greatest Problem": Religion and State Formation in Meiji Japan*. Cambridge, MA: Harvard University Asia Center, 2014.

Melling, Joseph, and Bill Forsythe, eds. *Insanity, Institutions and Society, 1800–1914: A Social History of Madness in Comparative Perspective*. London: Routledge, 1999.

Meyer, Manuella. *Reasoning against Madness: Psychiatry and the State in Rio de Janeiro, 1830–1944*. New York: University of Rochester Press, 2017.

Micale, Mark. *Approaching Hysteria: Disease and Its Interpretations*. Princeton, NJ: Princeton University Press, 1995.

Micale, Mark. *Hysterical Men: The Hidden History of Male Nervous Illness*. Cambridge, MA: Harvard University Press, 2008.

Micale, Mark. "On the 'Disappearance' of Hysteria: A Study in the Clinical Deconstruction of a Diagnosis." *Isis* 84, no. 3 (September 1993): 496–526.

Minas, Harry, and Hervita Diatri. "Pasung: Physical Restraint and Confinement of the Mentally Ill in the Community." *International Journal of Mental Health Systems* 2, no. 8 (2016). https://doi.org/10.1186/1752-4458-2-8.

Mitra, Durba. *Indian Sex Life: Sexuality and the Colonial Origins of Modern Social Thought.* Princeton, NJ: Princeton University Press, 2020.

Miyake, Yoshiko. "Doubling Expectations: Motherhood and Women's Factory Work under State Management in Japan in the 1930s and 1940s." In *Recreating Japanese Women, 1600–1945,* edited by Gail Lee Bernstein, 267–295. Berkeley: University of California Press, 1991.

Mooney, Graham, and Jonathan Reinarz, eds., *Permeable Walls: Historical Perspectives on Hospital and Asylum Visiting.* Amsterdam: Rodopi, 2009.

Moran, James. "Architectures of Madness: Informal and Formal Spaces of Treatment and Care in Nineteenth-Century New Jersey." In *Madness, Architecture, and the Built Environment: Psychiatric Spaces in Historical Context,* edited by Leslie Topp, James E. Moran, and Jonathan Andrews, 153–172. New York: Routledge, 2007.

Morita, Masatake. "Tosa ni okeru inugami ni tsuite." *Shinkeigaku zasshi* 3, no. 3 (1904): 129–130.

Moscucci, Ornella. *The Science of Woman: Gynaecology and Gender in England, 1800–1929.* Cambridge: Cambridge University Press, 1990.

Motō, Aki. "Sharukō no jidai to Miura Kinnosuke." *Rinshō shinkeigaku* 33 (1993): 1259–1264.

Munakata, Tsunetsugu. "Japanese Attitudes toward Mental Illness and Mental Health Care." In *Japanese Culture and Behavior,* edited by Takie Sugiyama Lebra and William P. Libra, 369–378. Honolulu: University of Hawai'i Press, 1986.

Muta, Kazue. "Images of the Family in Meiji Periodicals: The Paradox Underlying the Emergence of the 'Home." Translated by Marcella S. Gregory. *U.S.-Japan Women's Journal,* English supp. 7 (1994): 53–71.

Muta, Kazue. *Senryaku to shite no kazoku: kindai Nihon no kokumin kokka keisei to josei.* Tokyo: Shinyōsha, 1996.

Nagai, Junko. "Seishinbyōsha' to keihō dai sanjūkyūjyō no seiritsu." *Soshio saiensu* 11 (2005): 225–240.

Nagy, Margit. *"How Shall We Live?": Social Change, the Family Institution, and Feminism in Prewar Japan.* PhD diss., University of Washington, 1981.

Nagy, Margit. "Middle-Class Working Women during the Interwar Years." In *Recreating Japanese Women, 1600–1945,* edited by Gail Lee Bernstein, 199–216. Berkeley: University of California Press, 1991.

Nakamura, Eri. "Psychiatrists as Gatekeepers of War Expenditure: Diagnosis and Distribution of Military Pensions in Japan during the Asia-Pacific War." *East Asian Science, Technology, and Society* 13, no. 1 (2019): 57–75.

Nakamura, Karen. *A Disability of the Soul: An Ethnography of Schizophrenia and Mental Illness in Contemporary Japan.* Ithaca, NY: Cornell University Press, 2013.

Nakamura, Kokyō. *Hisuterii no ryōhō.* Tokyo: Shufu No Tomo Sha, 1932.

Nakamura, Kokyō. *Seishineisei kōwa.* 3 vols. Tokyo: Shufu No Tomo Sha, 1933.

Nakamura, Masaichi. "Ugetsu monogatari Kibitsu no kama kō: Shōtarō to zashikirō." *Shōkei gakuin kenkyū kiyō* 4 (2010): 17–28.

Nakamura, Miri. "The Cult of Happiness: Maid, Housewife, and Affective Labor in Higuchi Ichiyō's 'Warekara.'" *Journal of Japanese Studies* 41, no. 1 (Winter 2015): 45–78.

Nakamura, Osamu. *Rakuhoku Iwakura to seishiniryō: seishinbyō kanja kazokuteki kango no dentō no keisei to shōshitsu.* Tokyo: Sekai Shisōsha, 2013.

Nakamura, Teiri. *Kitsune no Nihon shi: Kinsei kindai hen.* Tokyo: Nihon Editā Sukūru Shuppanbu, 2003.

Nakatani, Yōji. "The Birth of Criminology in Modern Japan." In *Criminals and Their Scientists: The History of Criminology in International Perspective,* edited by Peter Becker and Richard D. Wetzell, 281–300. Cambridge: Cambridge University Press, 2009.

Nakatani, Yōji. "Seishinbyōsha kangohō wa naze seitei saretaka." *Seishin igakushi kenkyū* 5, no. 1 (2001): 181–197.

Nakayama, Izumi. *Periodic Struggles: Menstruation Leave in Japan.* PhD diss., Harvard University, 2007.

Newell, Susan. "Women Primary School Teachers and the State in Interwar Japan." In *Society and the State in Interwar Japan,* edited by Elise K. Tipton, 17–41. London and New York: Routledge, 1997.

Ninomiya, Shūhei. "Kindai koseki seido no kakuritsu to kazoku no tōsei." In *Koseki to mibun tōroku,* edited by Nobuyoshi Toshitani, Hiroshi Kamata, and Hiroshi Hiramatsu, 146–164. Tokyo: Waseda Daigaku Shuppanbu, 2005.

Nishida, Tomomi. *Chi no shisō: Edo Jidai no Shiseikan.* Tokyo: Kenseisha, 1995.

Nishihara, Haruo, ed. *Kyū keihō: Meiji 13-nen.* Tokyo: Shinzansha, 1994–1997.

Nishikawa, Kaoru. "Seishinbyōsha kangohō seitei ni kansuru ichikenkyū: seitei ito ni kansuru senkō kenkyū hihan." *Gendai shakai bunka kenkyū* 24 (2001): 143–160.

Nishikawa, Kaoru. "Soma jiken to seishinbyōsha kangōhō seitei no kanren: senkō kenkyū rebū." *Gendai shakai bunka kenkyū (Niigata daigaku daigakuin gendai shakai bunka kenkyūka)* 26 (2003): 35–51.

Nishikawa, Yūko. "The Changing Form of Dwellings and the Establishment of the Katei (Home) in Modern Japan." Translated by Manko Muro Yokokawa. *U.S.-Japan Women's Journal* English supp. 8 (1995): 3–36.

Nozoe, Atsuyoshi. *Josei to hanzai, Kindai hanzai kagaku zenshū.* Tokyo: Bukyōsha, 1930.

Oda, Makoto. *Sei.* Tokyo: Sanseidō, 1996.

Oda, Susumu, ed. *"Hentai shinri" to Nakamura Kokyō: Taishō bunka e no shinshikaku.* Tokyo: Fuji Shuppan, 2001.

Ogata, Koan. *Fushi keiken ikun.* 25 vols. Osaka: Akitayatemon, 1857.

Okada, Aoi, and Satomi Kurosu. "Succession and the Death of the Household Head in Early Modern Japan: A Case Study of a Northeastern Village, 1720–1870." *Continuity and Change* 13 (1998): 143–166.

Okada, Hajime, ed. *Haifū yanagidaru zenshū.* 12 vols. Tokyo: Sanseido, 1976.

Okada, Yasuo. *Nihon seishinka iryōshi.* Tokyo: Igaku Shoin, 2002.

Okada, Yasuo. "Shimamura Shun'ichi shōden: hiun no seishinbyōgakusha." *Nihon ishigaku zasshi* 38, no. 4 (1992): 603–634.

Okada, Yasuo. *Shisetsu Matsuzawa byōinshi: 1879–1980*. Tokyo: Iwasaki Gakujutsu Shuppansha, 1981.

Okada, Yasuo, Hashimoto, Akira, and Komine, Kazushige, eds. *Seishin shōgaisha mondai shiryō shūse*. 9 vols. Tokyo: Rikka Shuppan, 2010.

Ōkuda, Akiko. "Jochū no rekishi." In *Onna to otoko no jikū—Nihon joseishi saikō*, edited by Akiko Ōkuda, 5:376–410. Tokyo: Fujiwara Shoten, 1995.

Omata, Wa'ichirō. *Seishinbyōin no kigen: kindai hen*. Tokyo: Ōta Shuppan, 2000.

Oosterhuis, Harry. *Stepchildren of Nature: Krafft-Ebing, Psychiatry, and the Making of Sexual Identity*. Chicago: University of Chicago Press, 2000.

Otsubo, Sumiko. "Engendering Eugenics: Feminists and Marriage Restriction Legislation in the 1920s." In *Gendering Modern Japanese History*, edited by Barbara Molony and Kathleen S. Uno, 225–256. Cambridge, MA: Harvard University Asia Center, 2005.

Ozaki, Koji. "1879-nen korera to chihō eisei seisaku no tankan: Aichi-ken wo jirei to shite." *Nihonshi kenkyū* 418 (June 1997): 41–48.

Park, Jin-kyung. "Managing 'Dis-ease': Print Media, Medical Images, and Patent Medicine Advertisements in Colonial Korea." *International Journal of Cultural Studies* 21, no. 4 (2018): 420–439.

Parle, Julie. *States of Mind: Searching for Mental Health in Natal and Zululand, 1868–1918*. Scottsville, South Africa: University of KwaZulu-Natal Press, 2007.

Peng, Ito. "Social Care in Crisis: Gender, Demography, and Welfare State Restructuring in Japan." *Social Politics* 9, no. 3 (2002): 411–443.

Pflugfelder, Gregory. *Cartographies of Desire: Male-Male Sexuality in Japanese Discourse, 1600–1950*. Berkeley: University of California Press, 1999.

Pierce, Joseph M. *Argentine Intimacies: Queer Kinship in an Age of Splendor, 1890–1910*. Albany: State University of New York Press, 2019.

Pinto, Sarah. *Daughters of Parvati: Women and Madness in Contemporary India*. Philadelphia: University of Pennsylvania Press, 2014.

Prestwich, Patricia. "Family Strategies and Medical Power: 'Voluntary' Committal in a Parisian Asylum, 1876–1914." *Journal of Social History* 27 (1994): 799–818.

Quarshie, Nan Osei. "Contracted Intimacies: Psychiatric Nursing Conspiracies in the Gold Coast." *Politique africaine* 157 (2020): 91–110.

Ragsdale, Kathryn. "Marriage, the Newspaper Business, and the Nation-State: Ideology in the Late Meiji Serialized Katei Shōsetsu." *Journal of Japanese Studies* 24, no. 2 (Summer 1998): 229–255.

Reichert, Jim. *In the Company of Men: Representations of Male-Male Sexuality in Meiji Literature*. Stanford, CA: Stanford University Press, 2006.

Robertson, Jennifer. "Hemato-Nationalism: The Past, Present, and Future of 'Japanese Blood.'" *Medical Anthropology: Cross-Cultural Studies in Health and Illness* 21, no. 2 (2012): 93–112.

Robertson, Jennifer, and Gail Lee Bernstein. "Shingaku Woman: Straight from the Heart." In *Recreating Japanese Women, 1600–1945*, edited by Gail Lee Bernstein, 88–107. Berkeley: University of California Press, 1991.

Roden, Donald. "Taishō Culture and the Problem of Gender Ambivalence." In *Culture and Identity*, edited by Thomas Rimer, 37–56. Princeton, NJ: Princeton University Press, 1990.

Rogaski, Ruth. *Hygienic Modernity: Meanings of Health and Disease in Treaty-Port China*. Berkeley: University of California Press, 2004.

Röhl, Wilhelm, ed. *History of Law in Japan since 1868*. Leiden: Brill, 2005.

Rokuhara, Hiroko. "Local Officials and the Meiji Conscription Campaign." *Monumenta Nipponica* 60, no. 1 (2005): 81–110.

Rosenberger, Nancy. *Middle-aged Japanese Women and the Meanings of the Menopausal Transition*. PhD diss., University of Michigan, 1984.

Rosenberger, Nancy. "The Process of Discourse: Usages of a Japanese Medical Term." *Social Science and Medicine* 34 (1992): 237–247.

Rosenberger, Nancy. "Productivity, Sexuality, and Ideologies of Menopausal Problems in Japan." In *Health, Illness, and Medical Care in Japan: Cultural and Social Dimensions*, edited by Edward Norbeck and Margaret Lock, 158–188. Honolulu: University of Hawai'i Press, 1987.

Roth, Cassia. *A Miscarriage of Justice: Women's Reproductive Lives and the Law in Early Twentieth-Century Brazil*. Stanford, CA: Stanford University Press, 2020.

Rousseau, Julie. *Enduring Labors: The "New Midwife" and the Modern Culture of Childbearing in Early Twentieth Century Japan*. PhD diss., Columbia University, 1998.

Ruggiero, Kristin. "Honor, Maternity, and the Disciplining of Women: Infanticide in Late Nineteenth-Century Buenos Aires." *Hispanic American Historical Review* 72, no. 3 (1992): 353–373.

Ruggiero, Kristin. *Modernity in the Flesh: Medicine, Law, and Society in Turn-of-the-Century Argentina*. Stanford, CA: Stanford University Press, 2004.

Saito, Osamu. "Marriage, Family Labour and the Stem Family Household: Traditional Japan in a Comparative Perspective." *Continuity and Change* 15 (2000): 17–45.

Saito, Satoru. *Detective Fiction and the Rise of the Japanese Novel, 1880–1930*. Cambridge, MA: Harvard University Asia Center, 2012.

Saitō, Tamao. "Gunma-ken kanka seishinbyōsha shitaku kanchi jyōkyō shisatsu hōkoku." In *Seishin shōgaisha mondai shiryō shūse*, edited by Yasuo Okada, Akira Hashimoto, and Kazushige Komine, 4:43–65. Tokyo: Rikka Shuppan, 2010.

Sand, Jordan. *House and Home in Modern Japan: Architecture, Domestic Space, and Bourgeois Culture, 1880–1930*. Cambridge, MA: Harvard University Asia Center, 2003.

Sand, Jordan, and Steven Wills. "Governance, Arson, and Firefighting in Edo, 1600–1868." In *Flammable Cities: Urban Conflagration and the Making of the Modern World*, edited by Greg Bankoff, Uwe Luebken, and Jordan Sand, 44–62. Madison: University of Wisconsin Press, 2012.

Sasaoka, Shōzō. *Fujinbyōsha no kokoroe.* Tokyo: Self-published, 1910.

Sato, Barbara. *The New Japanese Woman: Modernity, Media, and Women in Interwar Japan.* Durham, NC: Duke University Press, 2003.

Satō, Masahiro. *Seishin shikkan gensetsu no rekishi shakaigaku: "Kokoro no yamai" wa naze ryūkō suru no ka.* Toyko: Shin'yōsha, 2013.

Sawada, Janine. *Practical Pursuits: Religion, Politics, and Personal Cultivation in Nineteenth-Century Japan.* Honolulu: University of Hawai'i Press, 2004.

Schmeiser, Susan R. "The Ungovernable Citizen: Psychopathy, Sexuality, and the Rise of Medico-Legal Reasoning." *Yale Journal of Legal History* 20, no. 2 (2008): 163–240.

Serizawa, Kazuya. *"Hō" kara kaihōsareru kenryoku: hanzai, kyōki, hinkon, soshite Taishō demokurashii.* Tokyo: Shinyōsha, 2001.

Shapiro, Ann-Louise. *Breaking the Code: Female Criminality in Fin-de-Siècle Paris.* Stanford, CA: Stanford University Press, 1996.

Shapiro, Hugh. "Pathologizing Marriage: Neuropsychiatry and the Escape of Women in Early Twentieth-Century China." In *Psychiatry and Chinese History*, edited by Howard Chiang, 129–141. London: Pickering and Chatto, 2014.

Shelton, Laura. "Bodies of Evidence: Honor, *Prueba Plena*, and Emerging Medical Discourses in Northern Mexico's Infanticide Trials in the Late Nineteenth and Early Twentieth Centuries." *Americas* 74, no. 4 (2017): 457–480.

Shigehisa, Kuriyama. "The Historical Origins of Katakori." *Japan Review* 9 (1997): 127–149.

Shikita, Minoru, and Shinchi Tsuchiya. *Crime and Criminal Policy in Japan: Analysis and Evaluation of the Showa Era, 1926–1988.* New York: Springer-Verlag, 1992.

Shimamura, Shun'ichi. "Shimane kenka kohyōbyō torishirabe hōkoku." In *Tōkyō Igakkai Zasshi* 6, no. 6 (1892): 1–18; 7, no. 3 (1893): 24–39. Reprinted in *Kindai shomin seikatsushi*, edited by Hiroshi Minami, 20:44–72. Tokyo: San'ichi Shobō, 1984–1988.

Shimazaki, Satoko. *Edo Kabuki in Transition: From the Worlds of the Samurai to the Vengeful Female Ghost.* New York: Columbia University Press, 2016.

Shimazaki, Tōson. *Before the Dawn.* Translated by William E. Naff. Honolulu: University of Hawai'i Press, 1987.

Shimazono, Susumu. *Iyasu chi no keifu: Kagaku to shūkyō no hasami.* Tokyo: Yoshikawa Kōbunkan, 2003.

Shimizu, Michiko. *"Jochū" imēji no katei bunkashi.* Tokyo: Sekai Shisōsha, 2004.

Shimizu, Shōjirō. *Meiji, Taishō, Shōwa norowareta josei hanzai.* Tokyo: Yoshie Shobō, 1965.

Shimoda, Mitsuzō, and Naoki Sugita. *Saishin seishinbyōgaku.* Tokyo: Kokuseidō Shoten, 1922.

Shinmura, Taku. *Nihon bukkyō no iryōshi.* Tokyo: Hōsei Daigaku Shuppan Kyoku, 2013.

Shinotsuka, Eiko. "Japanese Care Assistants in Hospitals, 1918–1988." In *Japanese Women Working*, edited by Janet Hunter, 149–180. London: Routledge, 1993.

Shiomitsu, Takashi. "Seishin shōgaisha no Kazoku seisaku ni kan suru ikkōsatsu: hogosha seidō no hensen wo tegakari ni." *Fukushi kyōiku kaihatsu sentaa kiyō* 13 (2017): 73–89.

Shirasugi, Etsuo. "Hieshō no hakken." In *Kindai Nihon no shintai kankaku*, edited by Shigehisa Kuriyama and Kazutoshi Kitazawa, 65–68. Tokyo: Seikyūsha, 2004.

Shorter, Edward. *A History of Psychiatry: From the Era of the Asylum to the Age of Prozac.* New York: John Wiley & Sons, 1997.

Showalter, Elaine. *The Female Malady: Women, Madness, and Culture in England, 1830–1980.* New York: Pantheon Books, 1985.

Showalter, Elaine. "Hysteria, Feminism, and Gender." In *Hysteria beyond Freud*, edited by Sander L. Gilman, Helen King, Roy Porter, G. S. Rousseau, and Elaine Showalter, 286–344. Berkeley: University of California Press, 1993.

Showalter, Elaine. *Hystories: Hysterical Epidemics and Modern Culture.* New York: Columbia University Press, 1997.

Shufu no tomo, 1912–1937.

Silver, Mark. *Purloined Letters: Cultural Borrowing and Japanese Crime Literature, 1868–1937.* Honolulu: University of Hawai'i Press, 2008.

Silverberg, Miriam. *Erotic Grotesque Nonsense: The Mass Culture of Japanese Modern Times.* Berkeley: University of California Press, 2006.

Simmons, Duane B. *Cholera Epidemics in Japan: With a Monograph on the Influence of the Habits and Customs of Races on the Prevalence of Cholera.* Shanghai: Statistical Department of the Inspectorate General of Customs, 1880.

Simonis, Fabien. *Mad Acts, Mad Speech, and Mad People in Late Imperial Chinese Law and Medicine.* PhD diss., Princeton University, 2010.

Smith, Robert J. "Making Village Women into 'Good Wives and Wise Mothers' in Prewar Japan." *Journal of Family History* 8, no. 1 (1983): 70–84.

Smith, Thomas C. *The Agrarian Origins of Modern Japan.* Stanford, CA: Stanford University Press, 1959.

Smith-Rosenberg, Carroll. "The Hysterical Woman: Sex Roles and Role Conflict in Nineteenth Century America." *Social Research* 39 (Winter 1972): 652–678.

Smith-Rosenberg, Carroll, and Charles Rosenberg. "The Female Animal: Medical and Biological Views of Woman and Her Role in Nineteenth-Century America." *Journal of American History* 60, no. 2 (1973): 332–356.

Smyers, Karen. *The Fox and the Jewel: Shared and Private Meaning in Contemporary Japanese Inari Worship.* Honolulu: University of Hawai'i Press, 1999.

Sone, Sachiko. "Japanese Coal Mining: Women Discovered." In *Women Miners in Developing Countries: Pit Women and Others*, edited by Kuntala Lahiri-Dutt and Martha Macintyre, 51–72. Aldershot; Burlington: Ashgate, 2006.

Stalker, Nancy K. *Kurozumikyō and the New Religions of Japan.* Honolulu: University of Hawai'i Press, 2007.

Steenstrup, Carl. A History of Law in Japan until 1868. Leiden: E. J. Brill, 1991.

Stevenson, Lisa. *Life beside Itself: Imagining Care in the Canadian Arctic.* Berkeley: University of California Press, 2014.

Sugie, Tadasu. *Hisuterii no kenkyū to sono ryōhō*. Tokyo: Shimada Bunseikan, 1915.

Sugiyama, Hiroshi. "Bunmei kaikaki no hayariyamai to minshū ishiki: Meiji jūnendai no korera matsuri to korera sōdō." *Machida shiritsu jiyū minken shiryōkan* 2 (1988): 19–50.

Suh, Jiyoung. "The Gaze on the Threshold: Korean Housemaids of Japanese Families in Colonial Korea." *positions* 27, no. 3 (2019): 437–468.

Suzuki, Akihito. "Between Two Psychiatric Regimes: Migration and Psychiatry in Early Twentieth-Century Japan." In *Migration, Ethnicity, and Mental Health: International Perspectives, 1840–2010*, edited by Angela McCarthy and Catharine Coleborne, 141–156. New York and London: Routledge, 2012.

Suzuki, Akihito. *Madness at Home: The Psychiatrist, the Patient, and the Family in England, 1820–1860*. Berkeley: University of California Press, 2006.

Suzuki, Akihito. "Psychiatric Hospitals, Domestic Strategies and Gender Issues in Tokyo c. 1920–1945." *History of Psychiatry* 33, no. 3 (Forthcoming 2022).

Suzuki, Akihito. "The State, Family, and the Insane in Japan, 1900–45." In *The Confinement of the Insane: International Perspectives, 1800–1965*, edited by Roy Porter and David Wright, 193–225. Cambridge: Cambridge University Press, 2003.

Suzuki, Akihito. "Voices of Madness in Japan: Narrative Devices at the Psychiatric Bedside and in Modern Literature." In *The Routledge History of Madness and Mental Health*, edited by Greg Eghigian, 245–260. London: Routledge, 2017.

Suzuki, Akihito. "Were Asylums Men's Places? Male Excess in the Asylum Population in Japan in the Early Twentieth Century." In *Psychiatric Cultures Compared: Psychiatry and Mental Health Care in the Twentieth Century*, edited by Marijke Gijswijt-Hofstra, Harry Oosterhuis, Joost Vijselaar, and Hugh Freeman, 295–311. Amsterdam: Amsterdam University Press, 2005.

Suzuki, Akihito, and Mika Suzuki. "Cholera, Consumer and Citizenship: Modernisations of Medicine in Japan." In *The Development of Modern Medicine in Non-Western Countries*, edited by Hormoz Ebrahimnejad, 184–203. London: Routledge, 2008.

Suzuki, Michiko. *Becoming Modern Women: Love and Female Identity in Prewar Japanese Literature and Culture*. Palo Alto, CA: Stanford University Press, 2009.

Suzuki, Tomi. *Narrating the Self: Fictions of Japanese Modernity*. Palo Alto, CA: Stanford University Press, 1996.

Suzuki, Zenji. *Nihon no yūseigaku*. Tokyo: Sankyō Shuppan, 1983.

Suzuki, Zenji, Matsubara, Yōko and Sakano, Tōru. "Yūseigaku-shi kenkyū no dōkō III: Amerika oyobi Nihon no yūseigaku ni kansuru rekishi kenkyū." *Kagakushi kenkyū* 34 (1995): 101–106.

Takahashi, Aya. *The Development of the Japanese Nursing Profession: Adopting and Adapting Western Influences*. London; New York: RoutledgeCurzon, 2004.

Takahashi, Masao. *Sōseki bungaku ga monogataru mono: shinkei suijakusha e no ikei to iyashi*. Tokyo: Misuzu Shobō, 2009.

Takahashi, Satoshi. *Bakumatsu orugi: korera ga yatte kita!* Tokyo: Asahi Shinbunsha, 2005.

Takashi, Katō. "Governing Edo." In *Edo and Paris: Urban Life and the State in the Early Modern Era*, edited by James L. MacClain, John M. Merriman, and Kaoru Ugawa, 41–67. Ithaca, NY: Cornell University Press, 1997.

Tamura, Kasaburō. *Shinkei no eisei*. Tokyo: Yomiuri Shinbunsha, 1907.

Tanaka, Hikaru. *Gekkei to hanzai: josei hanzai ron no shingi wo tou*. Tokyo: Hihyōsha, 2006.

Terazawa, Yuki. *Knowledge, Power, and Women's Reproductive Health in Japan, 1690–1945*. Cham: Palgrave Macmillan, 2018.

Thal, Sarah. *Rearranging the Landscape of the Gods: The Politics of a Pilgrimage Site in Japan, 1573–1912*. Chicago: University of Chicago Press, 2005.

Thal, Sarah. "Redefining the Gods: Politics and Survival in the Creation of Modern Kami." *Japanese Journal of Religious Studies* 29 (2002): 379–404.

Tipton, Elise K. "Pink Collar Work: The Café Waitress in Early Twentieth Century Japan." *Intersections: Gender, History and Culture in the Asian Context* 7 (March 2002). http://intersections.anu.edu.au/issue7/tipton.html.

Totman, Conrad. *Early Modern Japan*. Berkeley: University of California Press, 2005.

Trambaiolo, Daniel. "Native and Foreign in Tokugawa Medicine." *The Journal of Japanese Studies* 39, no. 2 (2013): 299–324.

Tsurumi, Patricia. *Factory Girls: Women in the Thread Mills of Meiji Japan*. Princeton, NJ: Princeton University Press, 1990.

Uchida, Ryūzō. *Tantei shōsetsu no shakaigaku*. Tokyo: Iwanami Shoten, 2001.

Ueda, Makoto, trans. *Light Verse from the Floating World: An Anthology of Premodern Japanese Senryū*. New York: Columbia University Press, 1999.

Ueno, Chizuko. *Kea no shakaigaku: tojisha shjken no fukushishakai e*. Tokyo: Ōta Shuppan, 2011.

Ueno, Chizuko. *Kindai kazoku no seiritsu to shūen*. Tokyo: Iwanami Shoten, 1994.

Umemori, Naoyuki. *Modernization through Colonial Mediations: The Establishment of the Police and Prison System in Meiji Japan*. PhD diss., University of Chicago, 2002.

Uno, Kathleen. "One Day at a Time: Work and Domestic Activities of Urban Lower-Class Women in Early Twentieth-Century Japan." In *Japanese Women Working*, edited by Janet Hunter, 37–68. London and New York: Routledge, 1993.

Uno, Kathleen. *Passages to Modernity: Motherhood, Childhood, and Social Reform in Early Twentieth-Century Japan*. Honolulu: University of Hawai'i Press, 1999.

Uno, Kathleen. "Questioning Patrilineality: On Western Studies of the Japanese Ie." *Positions* 4 (Winter 1996): 569–594.

Uno, Kathleen. "Womanhood, War, and Empire: Transmutations of 'Good Wife, Wise Mother' before 1931." In *Gendering Modern Japanese History*, edited by Barbara Molony and Kathleen Uno, 493–519. Cambridge, MA: Harvard University Asia Center, 2005.

Uno, Kathleen. "Women and Changes in the Household Division of Labor." In *Recreating Japanese Women, 1600–1945*, edited by Gail Lee Bernstein, 17–41. Berkeley: University of California Press, 1991.

Utsonomiya, Minori. "Seishinbyōsha kango hōan teishutsu ni itaru yōin ni kansuru kenkyū." *Shakai Jigyōshi Kenkyū* 36 (2009): 109–122.

Utsonomiya, Minori. "Seishinbyōsha kangohō no 'kango' gainen no kenshō." *Shakai Fukushigaku* 51, no. 3 (2010): 68.

Utsonomiya, Minori. "Seishinbyōsha kangohō seiritsuzen no seishin shōgaisha taisaku." *Tōkai Joshi Daigaku Kiyō* 26 (2006): 130–146.

Vaughan, Megan, and Sloan Mahone, eds. *Psychiatry and Empire*. Basingstoke: Palgrave Macmillan, 2007.

Veith, Ilza. *Hysteria: The History of a Disease*. Chicago: University of Chicago Press, 1965.

Vogel, Suzanne. *Professional Housewife: The Career of Urban Middle Class Japanese Women*. Cambridge, MA: Institute for Independent Study, Radcliffe College, 1988.

Wakabayashi, Misako, ed. *Berutsu nihon bunka ronshū*. Tokyo: Tōkai Daigaku Suppankai, 2001.

Waswo, Ann. "The Transformation of Rural Society, 1900–1950." In *The Cambridge History of Japan*, edited by John Whitney Hall et al., 6:539–605. Cambridge: Cambridge University Press, 1989.

Watarai, Yoshiichi. *Meiji no seishin isetsu: shinkeibyō shinkei suijaku kamigakari*. Tokyo: Iwanami Shoten, 2003.

Wetzell, Richard. "Criminology in Weimar and Nazi Germany." In *Criminals and Their Scientists: The History of Criminology in International Perspective*, edited by Peter Becker and Richard F. Wetzell, 401–424. Cambridge: Cambridge University Press, 2009.

Wetzell, Richard. *Inventing the Criminal: A History of German Criminology, 1880–1945*. Chapel Hill: University of North Carolina Press, 2000.

Williams, Duncan. *The Other Side of Zen: A Social History of Sōtō Zen Buddhism in Tokugawa Japan*. Princeton, NJ: Princeton University Press, 2004.

Winfield, Pamela D. "Curing with Kaji: Healing and Esoteric Empowerment in Japan." *Japanese Journal of Religious Studies* 32, no. 1 (2005): 107–130.

Wright, David. "Getting Out of the Asylum: Understanding the Confinement of the Insane in the Nineteenth Century." *Social History of Medicine* 10 (1997): 137–155.

Wright, Diana E. "Female Crime and State Punishment in Early Modern Japan." *Journal of Women's History* 16, no. 3 (2004): 10–29.

Wu, Harry Yi-Jui, and Wen-Ji Wang, eds. "Making and Mapping Psy Sciences in East and Southeast Asia." *East Asian Science, Technology, and Society* 10, no. 2 (June 2016): 109–120.

Wu, Yi-Li. *Reproducing Women: Medicine, Metaphor, and Childbirth in Late Imperial China*. Berkeley: University of California Press, 2010.

Wu, Yu-chuan. *A Disorder of Ki: Alternative Treatments for Neurasthenia in Japan, 1890–1945*. PhD diss., University College London, 2012.

Yamagami, Akira. "Seishin kantei—sono rekishiteki hensen to shomondai." *Seishin igaku* 41, no. 10 (1999): 1032–1042.

Yamaguchi, Tomomi. "The Mainstreaming of Feminism and the Politics of Backlash in Twenty-First-Century Japan." In *Rethinking Japanese Feminisms*, edited by Julia C. Bullock, Ayako Kano, and James Walker, 68–85. Honolulu: University of Hawai'i Press, 2017.

Yamanaka, Einosuke. "Merchant 'House' (Iye) and Its Succession in Kyoto during the Tokugawa Era." *Osaka University Law Review* 11 (1963): 47–58.

Yamano, Haruo, and Narita, Ryūichi. "Minshū bunka to nashonarizumu." In *Kōza Nihonshi*, edited by Kenkyūkai Rekishigaku and Kenkyūkai Nihonshi, 9:253–292. Tokyo: Daigaku Shuppankai, 1985.

Yamashita, Mai. *Kangofu no rekishi: yorisou senmonshoku no tanjō*. Tokyo: Yoshikawa Kōbunkan, 2017.

Yamazaki, Tasuku. "Seishinbyōsha shogukō 4." *Shinkeigaku zashi* 34 (1932): 399–412.

Yomiuri shinbun, 1874–1937.

Yanagita, Kunio. *Japanese Manners and Customs in the Meiji Era*. Translated by Charles S. Terry. Tokyo: Ōbunsha, 1957.

Yang, Timothy. *A Medicated Empire: The Pharmaceutical Industry and Modern Japan*. Ithaca, NY: Cornell University Press, 2021.

Yoo, Theodore Jun. *It's Madness: The Politics of Mental Health in Colonial Korea*. Berkeley: University of California Press, 2016.

Yoshida, Morio. *Tantei shōsetsu to nihon kindai*. Tokyo: Seikyūsha, 2004.

Yoshida, Teigo. "Mystical Retribution, Spirit Possession, and Social Structure in a Japanese Village." *Ethnology* 6 (July 1967): 237–262.

Yoshida, Teigo. *Nihon no tsukimono: shakai jinruigakuteki kōsatsu*. Tokyo: Chūō Kōronsha, 1974.

Yoshida, Teigo. "Spirit Possession and Village Conflict." In *Conflict in Japan*, edited by Ellis S. Krauss, Thomas Rohlen, and Patricia Steinhoff, 85–104. Honolulu: University of Hawai'i Press, 1984.

Yoshinaga, Shin'ichi. "The Birth of Japanese Mind Cure Methods." In *Religion and Psychotherapy in Modern Japan*, edited by Christopher Harding, Fumiaki Iwata, and Shin'ichi Yoshinaga, 76–102. London: Routledge, 2015.

Young, W. Evan. "Domesticating Medicine: The Production of Familial Knowledge in Nineteenth-Century Japan." *Historia Scientiarum* 27, no. 2 (2018): 127–149.

Young, W. Evan. *Family Matters: Managing Illness in Late Tokugawa Japan, 1750–1868*. PhD diss., Princeton University, 2015.

Index

For the benefit of digital users, indexed terms that span two pages (e.g., 52–53) may, on occasion, appear on only one of those pages.

Note: Page numbers followed by f indicate a figure on the corresponding page.

Printed in the USA
CPSIA information can be obtained
at www.ICGtesting.com
CBHW070709220124
3636CB00004B/6